THE HEALTH OF PRISONERS

THE WELLCOME INSTITUTE SERIES IN THE HISTORY OF MEDICINE

Forthcoming Titles

Warm Climates and Western Medicine
Edited by David Arnold

Metropolitan Maternity: Maternal and Infant Welfare Services in Early Twentieth Century London
Lara Marks

Marshall Hall: 1790–1857: Science and Medicine in Early Victorian Society
Diana Manuel

The History of Concepts of Contagion
Edited by W. F. Bynum and Bernadino Fantini

Academic enquiries regarding the series should be addressed to the editors W. F. Bynum and Roy Porter at the Wellcome Institute for the History of Medicine, 183 Euston Road, London NW1 2BE, UK

THE HEALTH OF PRISONERS

HISTORICAL ESSAYS

Edited by
Richard Creese, W. F. Bynum and J. Bearn

Rodopi

Amsterdam - Atlanta, GA 1995

First published in 1995
by Editions Rodopi B. V., Amsterdam – Atlanta, GA 1995.

Design and Typesetting by Christine Lavery, the Wellcome Trust.
Printed and bound in The Netherlands by Editions Rodopi B. V.,
Amsterdam – Atlanta, GA 1995.

British Library Cataloguing in Publication Data
A catalogue record for this book is available from the British Library
ISBN 90-5183-817-4 (Bound)

Health
The Health of Prisoners: Historical Essays – Amsterdam – Atlanta,
GA Rodopi. – ill.
(Clio Medica 34/The Wellcome Institute Series in the
History of Medicine)

CIP-GEGEVENS KONINKLIJKE BIBLIOTHEEK, DEN HAAG

Front cover: Wood engraving of Coldbath Fields Prison, from
Henry Mayhew and John Binny, *The criminal prisons of London*,
London: Charles Griffin, Bohn and Company, 1862.
(photograph: *Wellcome Institute Library, London*)

Met index lit. opg.
ISBN 90-5183-817-4 (Bound)
Trefw.: geneeskunde; geschiedenis; gevangenis wezen.

Printed in The Netherlands

Contents

Preface vi

Notes on Contributors vii

Introduction 1

1. Howard's Beginning: Prisons, Disease, Hygiene
Roy Porter 5

2. Medical Treatment and Prisoners' Health in Stafford Gaol during the Eighteenth Century
A. J. Standley 27

3. The Health of Prisoners and the Two Faces of Benthamism
Martin J. Wiener 44

4. Development of the Prison Medical Service, 1774–1895
Anne Hardy 59

5. Elizabeth Fry and Mid-Nineteenth Century Reform
Anne Summers 83

6. The Prison Medical Service and the Deviant 1895–1948
Joe Sim 102

7. Prison Doctors and Prison Suicide Research
Alison Liebling and Tony Ward 118

8. Health Services for Prisoners: Lost in Ambiguities
Richard Smith 134

9. The Criminal Lunatic Asylum System Before and After Broadmoor
Sir Louis Blom-Cooper 151

10. The Woolf Report and After
Stephen Tumim 163

11. The Lessons of History
Stephen Shaw 171

Index 177

Preface

This volume is the result of a Symposium held on 3 March 1993 at the Royal Society of Medicine. It was jointly sponsored by the Section of the History of Medicine of the RSM and the Wellcome Institute for the History of Medicine, and brought together historians, criminologists and many distinguished individuals actively involved in contemporary dimensions of prisoners' health. The papers generated a lively discussion which was recorded. Dr Creese went through the recordings and has transcribed portions where additional useful comment was made on the various themes which the Symposium threw up. These sections give the volume an unusual immediacy and confirm the topicality of historical inquiry into the health of prisoners.

The editors would like to thank those who have helped to bring both the Symposium and this volume into being, especially Nechama Lewis of the Royal Society of Medicine, Sally Bragg of the Wellcome Institute, and Christine Lavery of the Publishing Department of the Wellcome Trust.

Notes on Contributors

Joe Bearn is a former Senior Lecturer in Anatomy at The Middlesex Hospital Medical School. He was Vice-President of the Section of the History of Medicine at the Royal Society of Medicine 1979–1982.

Sir Louis Blom-Cooper QC was called to the Bar in 1952. He was joint Director of the Legal Research Unit at Bedford College 1967–82, and Visiting Professor of Law at Queen Mary College 1983–1988. He has published on many aspects of law and penal reform, and has been Vice-President of the Howard League for Penal Reform since 1984.

W. F. Bynum is Director of the Academic Unit at the Wellcome Institute for the History of Medicine and Professor of History of Medicine in the University of London. He is General Editor of the Wellcome Institute for the History of Medicine Series (with Roy Porter) and, since 1980, has been Co-Editor of the quarterly journal *Medical History*. Recent publications include (joint editor with Roy Porter): *Companion Encyclopedia of the History of Medicine* (London: Routledge, 1993) and *Science and the Practice of Medicine in the Nineteenth Century* (Cambridge: Cambridge University Press, 1994).

Richard Creese was Professor of Physiology at St Mary's Hospital Medical School from 1968 to 1982. He was President of the Section of the History of Medicine of the Royal Society of Medicine during 1992–93.

Anne Hardy is a lecturer at the Wellcome Institute for the History of Medicine. She has published several articles on disease and public health in the eighteenth and nineteenth centuries, and is the author of *The Epidemic Streets: Infectious Disease and the Rise of Preventive Medicine 1856–1900* (Oxford: Clarendon Press, 1993).

Alison Liebling is a Senior Research Associate at the Institute of Criminology, Cambridge, and a Research Fellow at Trinity Hall. Her publications include *Suicides in Prison* (London: Routledge, 1992) and *Suicide Attempts in Male Prisons* (London: Home Office, 1993) and she co-edited (with Tony Ward) *Deaths in Custody: International Perspectives* (London: Whiting & Birch, 1994).

Roy Porter is Professor of the Social History of Medicine at the Wellcome Institute for the History of Medicine. He is currently working on the history of gout. Recent books include *Mind Forg'd Manacles. Madness in England from the Restoration to the Regency* (London: Athlone, 1987); *A Social History of Madness* (London: Weidenfeld and Nicolson, 1987); *In Sickness and in Health. The British Experience, 1650–1850* (London: Fourth Estate, 1988); *Patient's Progress* (Oxford: Polity, 1989) – these last two co-authored with Dorothy Porter; *Health for Sale. Quackery in England 1660–1850* (Manchester: Manchester University Press, 1989) and *London: A Social History* (London: Hamish Hamilton, 1994).

Stephen Shaw has been Director of the Prison Reform Trust since 1981. Previously, he worked for the Home Office Research Unit and for the National Association for the Care and Resettlement of Offenders.

His current research interests include private sector involvement in the prison system, and Prison Service management. He is the author of a wide range of booklets and articles and edits the Prison Reform Trust magazine *Prison Report.*

Joe Sim is Professor of Criminology in the School of Social Sciences, Liverpool John Moores University. He is the author of *Medical Power in Prisons* (Milton Keynes: Open University Press, 1990); co-author (with Mike Fitzgerald) of *British Prisons* (Oxford: Blackwell, 1982); and co-author (with Phil Scraton and Paula Skidmore) of *Prisons Under Protest* (Milton Keynes: Open University Press, 1991).

Richard Smith is Editor of the *BMJ*, Chief Executive Officer of the BMJ Publishing Group, and Special Professor of Medical Journalism in the University of Nottingham. He has written and broadcast on a wide range of topics, and is the author of *Prison Health Care* (London: BMJ Publishing Group, 1984).

A. J. Standley's interest in prison history began when he was working at Chelmsford Prison in 1972 and was asked to reply to a letter received from a schoolboy seeking a brochure on the prison's past. He retired from the Prison Service at Stafford, in 1988, and has retained his interest. Most of his writings have been for the benefit of school students and have been deposited at the William Salt Library, Stafford.

Anne Summers is a Curator in the Department of Manuscripts of the British Library. Her *Angels and Citizens: British Women as Military Nurses 1854–1914* was published by Routledge in 1988. She is currently working on a study of women, religion and politics in Britain 1800–1930.

His Honour **Judge Stephen Tumim** was called to the Bar in 1955. He has been Chief Inspector of Prisons for England and Wales since 1987 and is presently Chairman of the British Art Market Standing Committee, President of the Royal Literary Fund, and Chairman of the Koestler Award Trust. His publications include *Great Legal Disasters* (London: Arthur Barker, 1983) and *Great Legal Fiascos* (London: Arthur Barker, 1985).

Tony Ward is Lecturer in Law at De Montfort University Leicester, and a former Co-Director of INQUEST, an organization which works with the relatives of people who die in custody. He is co-author (with Mick Ryan) of *Privatization and the Penal System* (Milton Keynes: Open University Press, 1989) and a contributor to *Legal Medicine in History* (eds M. J. Clarke and C. Crawford, Cambridge: Cambridge University Press, 1994). He co-edited (with Alison Liebling) *Deaths in Custody: International Perspectives* (London: Whiting & Birch, 1994), and is working on a study of the psychiatric aspects of criminal justice since 1880.

Martin J. Wiener, Jones Professor of History at Rice University, is the author of *Between Two Worlds: The Political Thought of Graham Wallas* (Oxford: Clarendon Press, 1971), *English Culture and the Decline of the Industrial Spirit 1850–1914* (Cambridge/New York: Cambridge University Press, 1981), and *Reconstructing the Criminal: Culture, Law and Policy in England 1830–1914* (Cambridge/New York: Cambridge University Press, 1990). He is currently writing a book on the meanings of violence in nineteenth - and twentieth-century Britain.

Introduction

The decade opened with the riots at Strangeways and elsewhere (April 1990), and in the subsequent report the question was posed as to why the riots did not happen earlier (Woolf Report 1991). The report was followed by a series of articles to the press on the iniquities of our prisons (*Times* 1 October 1991), on the unreformed prison medical service (*Independent* 29 April 1991) and on the endeavours of Ministers and officials to overhaul our antiquated and expensive penal system.

The Joint Symposium was arranged by the Section of the History of Medicine of the Royal Society of Medicine and by the Wellcome Institute for the History of Medicine. The term 'Health' in the title has been interpreted widely, and we have adopted wherever possible a historical approach in an endeavour to give perspective to problems which do not go away. It was planned to limit the topics to those from the end of the eighteenth century, in the United Kingdom, but at the close of the Symposium the researches of A.J. Standley on the medical treatment of prisoners in Staffordshire in the eighteenth century and earlier became available, and with the addition of his article the historical time-span has been extended to three centuries.

The series opens with Roy Porter on John Howard and his contemporaries. Howard's book on England's prisons was first published in 1777: the record is stark and compelling, and has survived both hagiography and debunking, and serves to open the great debate. After Standley's contribution on the jails of Staffordshire, there follow three papers which illustrate what happened in the nineteenth century, in which the haphazard and mindless savageries of Howard's time were replaced by an institutionalized system which in turn revealed and developed its own problems. Martin Wiener offers a perspective from Texas on the multitudinous activities and pervasive influence of Jeremy Bentham and his troops of followers; Anne Hardy relates the development of medical services which followed the establishment of the Victorian penal structure and the tensions which arose between the medical and disciplinary aspects of the work of the full-time medical officers, and she gives a considered assessment of the charge which would categorize the medical officers as part of a repressive apparatus of control. Anne Summers comments on the moving story of Elizabeth Fry and her experiences in a male dominated society.

Joe Sim has produced an analytical paper based on the theoretical model of Foucault and his followers in which history since the Gladstone Report of 1895 is used to illustrate the received framework. Sim gives poignant examples of the repression and degradation which in practice continued in the half-century which followed the efforts of the reformers and which extended the powers of medical personnel in prisons, and the implications must bear on the current debate on the administrative means for the delivery of health care in the penitentiary.

Alison Liebling and Tony Ward write on suicide in prisons, with the message that suicide is to be regarded not primarily as a medical matter but the responsibility of all who form an environment in which suicide is seen by some inmates as the only solution.

Although the delivery of health care may be expected to have only marginal effects on health, it would seem important to overhaul the prison medical service (now styled 'health care for prisons'), whose deficiencies have been listed in the article by Judge Tumim. Richard Smith and other commentators would remove the service from the Home Office and make it a part of the National Health Service, although Judge Tumim warns about the addition of new loads to the travailing NHS. Throughout the discussion of this and other topics it is remarkable how certain themes reappear, sometimes in new guises. The recurrent public alarm induced by increase in the perception of crime is documented by the Prison Reform Trust (1993). Jails were run in a casual manner for private profit in Howard's time, then absorbed into the centralized Victorian penal system, and some may now be privatised in an apparent attempt to change the nature of the management; overcrowding in prisons waxed in the late eighteenth century, waned with the convict prisons, grew intolerably in the decades following the Second World War, began to show some diminution with the efforts of the Home Office in the late 1980s, and has recently swollen again with the rhetoric of Home Secretaries who echo public apprehensions of the extent of crime.

We have from Richard Smith a contribution which is analytical and which faces the central problem of the aims and objects of the penal system. If the essential purpose may be recognized as condemnatory and hence retributive – with the theatrical and rhetorical aspects as essential ingredients of the criminal justice system – then the other rationalizations may be regarded as problematic. There are a few (but important) offenders whose detention serves to protect the public. Deterrence is refuted by the figures for reconviction. And indeed our prisons are considered to encourage and nurture a criminal culture; the notion that our present prisons can reform has ceased to have serious defenders.

This is followed by the historical contribution from Louis Blom-Cooper which details the changing concepts and success and failures of attempts to contain and care for the numerous heterogenous population of the mentally disordered.

Judge Tumim presents his thoughts on the manifold defects in the provision of health care, and Stephen Shaw gives a perspective on 200 years of conflict and change in the prison scene.

Whatever view we may take of the social purpose of the penal system, there can be no valid reason for British prisons to have the reputation of being squalid, brutalizing and smelly. They are also hideously expensive and the reconviction rate makes them poor value for money. From the multitude of reports and proposals which recur down the decades it would seem that the officials face some very formidable obstacles in attempting to respond, and this leads to speculation on the factors which may be responsible. These are complex but can be gleaned from Part II of the Woolf Report (1991). And if there is one issue of central importance it is that of overcrowding in prisons. The Woolf Report gives the view of the Director-General of the prison services in that it was his belief:

> that the life and work of the Prison Service have for the last 20 years been distorted by the problem of overcrowding. That single factor has dominated prisoners' lives ... it has skewed managerial effort and it has directed managerial effort away from positive developments. The removal of overcrowding is, in my view, an indispensable precondition of sustained and universal improvement in prison conditions.

Select Bibliography

Committee of Inquiry Into the United Kingdom Prison Services 1979 (May Report), London: HMSO.

Howard, J., *1777: The State of the Prisons* (London: J.M. Dent, Everyman Library, 1929).

Howard League, Press Information, February 1994.

Ignatieff, M., *A Just Measure of Pain* (Harmondsworth: Penguin Books, 1989).

Linebaugh, P., *The London Hanged: Crime and Civic Society in the Eighteenth Century* (London: Allen Lane, 1991).

Prison Disturbances April 1990, Report of an Enquiry by the Right Hon Lord Justice Woolf and His Honour Judge Stephen Tumim (London: HMSO, 1991).

Prison Reform Trust, *Trends in Juvenile Crime and Punishment*, Juvenile Justice Paper, 4 February 1993.

Rollin, H. R., *The Mentally Abnormal Offender and the Law* (London: Pergamon Press, 1969).

Rollin, H. R., *Festina Lente: A Psychiatric Odyssey* (London: The British Medical Journal, 1990).

Sim, J., *Medical Power in Prisons* (Milton Keynes: Open University Press, 1990).

Smith, R., *Prison Health Care* (London: British Medical Association, 1984).

Tumim S., *What are Prisons For? The Nicholas Bacon Memorial Lecture* (London: Daunt Books, 1991).

West, R., 'The Strangeways of Bentham,' *Spectator*, 7 April 1990, 20–22.

Wiener, M., *Reconstructing the Criminal: Culture, Law and Policy in England, 1830–1914* (Cambridge: Cambridge University Press, 1990).

1

Howard's Beginning: Prisons, Disease, Hygiene

Roy Porter
Wellcome Institute for the History of Medicine

'I could willingly spit upon his statue', was Charles Lamb's verdict on John Howard.[1] The Christian philanthropist has always stirred strong feelings, but chiefly they have been positive, verging on idolatry; and his martyr's death in 1790 of camp fever contracted visiting a Russian hospital doubtless did nothing to sully the odour of sanctity. As early as 1780, William Hayley had composed a panegyric *Ode to Howard* with a frontispiece designed by Romney. Erasmus Darwin eulogized the benefactor to humanity in his *Botanic Garden* (1791), and William Leslie Bowles chipped in with *Verses to John Howard* (1789) and *The Grave of Howard* (1790). Alongside the statue erected in St Paul's, at least three anonymous lives appeared shortly after his death, and the canonization process culminated in 1818 with James Baldwin Brown's *Memoir of the Public and Private Life of John Howard, Philanthropist.*[2] The moral fable of one who literally gave his life to inventing prison reform, *ex nihilo* so to speak, evidently carried great emotional charge. 'The history of prison science begins with Howard', pronounced Hepworth Dixon in 1850.[3] Over a hundred years later, a Home Secretary, the Rt Hon. Merlyn Rees, was still singing the old familiar songs of praise:

> The great virtue of John Howard's work was not only that he drew attention to the scandalous conditions in which prisoners were then housed, but that he did so at a time when there was little or no interest in prisons.[4]

Quite the reverse; I hope to show that far from being a solitary reformer a prophet crying in the wilderness, Howard was on a wave for prison reform, itself part of the late-Enlightenment tide of opinion impatient to reconstruct all manner of institutions – gaols, mad-houses, barracks, orphanages, workhouses, hospitals – to meet the needs of modernity. Howard himself generously acknowledged the work of 'the ingenious Dr Lind', of Stephen Hales, John Haygarth, John Fothergill, Sir John Pringle, John Coakley Lettsom, and many Continental confrères.[5]

As the Howard myth mushroomed, extraordinary achievements were laid at his feet. 'In eradicating typhus from English prisons', writes Leona Baumgartner, 'he was responsible for a medical achievement of no mean character', for his labours 'led not only to the immediate reform of these evils by legislative action, but to a wider social awakening which ultimately grew into those organized medical, sanitary and social activities which we now refer to as the public health movement'.[6] The former of these claims – Howard annihilated typhus – is patently incorrect. The latter – that he fathered the public health movement – is specious Whig history; not surprisingly it grew up in the historical *apologiae* of Victorian sanitarians fishing for famous forebears and iconoclastically eager to replace 'John Howard, Dissenter, Christian Philanthropist and Martyr' with a more congenial image: 'John Howard, Medical Officer of Health *avant la lettre*'.[7] But if Howard has been venerated, he has also, as we have seen, been vilified. Charles Lamb hated Howard, because he supposedly behaved like a martinet to his only son, locking him up in solitary confinement till he grew deranged enough to need formal confinement in Dr Arnold's Leicester Lunatic Asylum.[8] Thomas Carlyle, normally a fervent hero-worshipper, took exception to the do-gooder in Howard (he was, grumbled the peevish Scot, 'the innocent cause ... of the Benevolent-Platform Fever').[9] And a few recent psychohistorians have prodded around in the unconscious of that austere vegetarian and puritanical teetotaller evidently obsessed with filth, stench and punishment, a man whose prison reforms might, moreover, be cynically interpreted as contrived to serve not the inmates but rather the interests of an emergent industrializing order through the reinforcement of corrective discipline and thus social control.[10]

Though the man thus invites conflicting interpretations, the basic facts are fairly clear.[11] Born in 1726 the son of a London Dissenter, his father's death left Howard a rich young man. Buying himself an estate at Cardington in Bedfordshire, he threw himself into the role of improving landowner, rebuilding the labourers' cottages and generally encouraging efficiency and order. And in 1756 he had a personal taste of imprisonment when, voyaging to Lisbon to inspect the tragic effects of the celebrated earthquake, his ship was seized by privateers, and he was held in a dungeon in Brest till he could be ransomed. Hence he was well prepared to make reforming use of his time and office when, in 1773 at the age of 47, he was appointed High Sheriff of Bedfordshire. Appalled to discover that at Bedford gaol, thanks to the private enterprise system then operating, remand prisoners who had been acquitted nevertheless often remained under lock-and-key because they couldn't meet the keeper's fees, he began to visit the gaols of neighbouring counties to investigate their management.[12] Making inspection tours of prisons and infirmaries thereafter became the *raison d'être* of his life, major expeditions, at home and abroad, occupying much of 1774–6, 1781, 1783, 1785–6. Accompanied by his faithful attendant, John Prole, Howard allegedly travelled upwards of fifty thousand miles, notebook in hand, visiting prisons, hospitals, lazarettos, schools, and workhouses, interrogating the authorities, taking copies of the regulations, measuring the rooms, weighing the loaves and nibbling the provisions. Long before publication of his *magna opera*, Howard won renown as a prison expert. In March 1774 he gave evidence before the House of Commons in committee, being formally thanked for 'the humanity and zeal which have led him to visit the several gaols of this kingdom, and to communicate to the House the interesting observations he has made on that subject' (whether he tested the 'epidemic constitution' in the Chamber is not recorded).[13] In the 1774 session, two bills were passed, one for the abolition of certain gaolers' fees (14 Geo. III, c.20) – Howard's original crusade – and the other for improving the sanitary state of prisons and the better preservation of the health of the prisoners. This latter, popularly known as the Health of Prisoners Act (14 Geo. III c.59), empowered Justices of the Peace to intervene in prison administration to ensure health standards.[14] Magistrates could command the scrubbing and whitewashing of walls as well as the provision of sick-rooms, adequate ventilation and regular washing and cleaning facilities. The statute also authorized them for the first time to pay 'an experienced Surgeon or Apothecary' out of the rates, his responsibility being to report on the health of the prisoners (as Howard found, only a few gaols then had surgeons). Introduced by the Member for Taunton, the driving force behind this legislation was obviously Howard, who briefly harboured parliamentary ambitions, and he had copies of these acts printed at his personal expense and sent to the keeper of every county gaol in the country. One may guess that his subsequent prison peregrinations in the mid-1770s were undertaken largely to gauge their uptake and impact. In this, he must have been disappointed. In only fifteen out of 130 institutions he visited had the statutes been properly honoured.

Thereafter, Howard's life was one extended gaol and hospital grand tour, punctuated by the production of his two masterpieces, the *State of the Prisons in England and Wales*, which came out in

1777 with revised editions in 1780 and 1784, and then *An Account of the Principal Lazarettos in Europe: With Various Papers Relative to the Plague* (1789) – and a few lesser works besides.[15] But though Howard published extensively, he remains somewhat enigmatic. Austere and buttoned-up, without small-talk or bosom buddies, he lived an exceedingly disciplined life and seems never to have poured out his soul (the contrast with Elizabeth Fry is total). His detached prose and array of facts and figures provided shield his innermost thoughts, feelings and fantasies. Some, of course, have liked to see him as a straightforward, down-to-earth, no-nonsense figure. He came, he saw, he reported, he reformed. The 'science' of prison improvement, judged Hepworth Dixon,

> is almost solely attributable to Howard, and the method which he adopted.... He entered the prison perfectly untrammelled by previous notions. No false knowledge impeded his progress. He had no hypotheses to support – no pet crotchets to warp his judgement. Happily, too, he was not embarrassed by the refinements of legal learning. The evils which he saw he proposed to remedy in the most simple and unstatesmanlike fashion. If he found captives starving, he proposed that they should be fed; if sick, tended; if in irons, unmanacled; if unjustly detained, set free, – and so forth. With a sublime unconsciousness of the complicated difficulties, moral, social and political, which beset the question of criminal treatment in the minds of mere reasoners, Howard always accepted the obvious and common-sense view of the case.[16]

This fantasy of Howard the awfully English humane empiricist with an open mind and utter faith in the sovereignty of facts clearly will not do – Howard doubtless saw grievances through eyes primed in philosophy, moral theology and science. But his Dissenters' self-effacement has left him a kind of invisible man, Mr Inspector, the man behind a mask. While the impenetrability of the public persona causes problems, it may not, however, be entirely without compensations. For it encourages one to cast Howard as a representative figure of the times, an almost automatic agent of the protocols of surveillance, order and punishment that Foucault, Ignatieff and others have seen silently, surreptitiously on the march, forging modern disciplinary society.[17]

And however unfathomable, Howard remains a colossus and hence a suitable figure upon whom to target the key questions regarding pre-nineteenth-century prison and physic. We must sweep away the myths, avoiding both hagiography and demonology, neither kissing nor spitting upon the statue. We must look afresh. Was he chiefly a religious reformer? A humanitarian? A utilitarian? A sanitarian? Was it medicine or morality that moved him to act? Through what ideological lenses did he analyse the state of the prisons? What institutional utopia fired his imagination? Was Howard's end essentially in line with the designs of contemporaries who were cleaning up camps and ships, hulks and hospitals, bridewells and houses of correction? Or was there a singular Howardian twist, as with the scandalous panopticon that sprang from Bentham's haunted head?[18]

Big questions. And doubly difficult to answer. For, despite recent attention to early prison history,[19] all too little is known about Howard's henchmen, the supporting cast of prison reformers, architects and medics, men like William Blackburn, Howard's admirer and pupil, and the first British architect to specialize in the planning of prisons, tragically cut down when only forty in 1790, or James Neild, or John Mason Good.[20] Likewise, wider historical perspectives are still lacking. Howard, we know, travelled extensively; he extolled the Dutch rasp-houses and spin-houses as models for imitation. Yet, despite the pioneering work of Peter Spierenberg, we remain largely unaware how far late-Enlightenment prison reform in England paralleled or diverged from that pursued on the Continent.[21]

Howard recorded the shocking facts. The *State of the Prisons* is a melancholy chronicle of damp, dark, dank, airless cells, famished prisoners, negligent authorities, apathy, corruption, disease and death. Sometimes the brevity of the litany speaks for itself: 'The rooms too small and close; no yard; no water; no straw'. So much for Lichfield gaol.[22] On to Hereford: 'No fire-place: offensive sewers: no court: no water: no stated allowance: no employment'.[23] And then to Gloucester, where prisoners were locked in the castle. This was in a woeful state; it had but one court for all prisoners – only one day-room for males and females. The debtors' ward had no windows (keepers blocked them up, to evade window-tax), and a hole had been forced in the plaster wall, to let in light. The night-room for male felons was gloomy and the floor too ruinous to be mopped. The whole prison was greatly out of repair, and it had not been whitewashed for years. Many inmates had perished in it the previous year – due, it was said, to fever bred by a great dunghill piled up directly opposite the stairs leading up to the sleeping-area. The keeper had no salary, the debtors no food allowance. The former lived on extortion, the latter on charity.[24] The gaols in Shrewsbury, Stafford and Salisbury, Swansea and Southwark displayed minor variations, but the basic theme was everywhere the same: the system was rotten. At Exeter the felons' gaol for the county of Devonshire was the private property of an individual, John Denny

Rolle, whose family had held it for generations on grant from the Duchy of Cornwall. The Rolle family received from the gaol an annual income of £22 a year handed over by the keeper. The keeper in turn had to find this sum out of the profits he could squeeze out of the prisoners' fees and the prison 'tap', that is, the sale of beer. The result was all too predictable. The night dungeons, though not especially subterranean, were close, cramped and dismal; the windows small, and the whole very unhealthy. An infirmary had been built – that in itself was a little unusual – but it couldn't be used because the steps leading up to it were in a parlous state; and Howard was unblushingly informed by the surgeon that he was excused by contract from attending any prisoner in the cells sick of the gaol fever![25] Wise fellow, for the gaol fever was a killer. 'The prison is a room, or passage, $23^1/2$ feet by $7^1/2$, with only one small window, and three dungeons, or cages, on the side opposite' – this is Launceston in Cornwall:

> these are about $6^1/2$ feet deep; one 9 feet long, one about 8; one not 5. This last for women. They were all very offensive; no chimney; no water; no sewers; damp earth floors; no infirmary. The court not secure, and prisoners seldom permitted to go out to it. Indeed the whole prison is out of repair, and yet the gaoler lives distant. I once found the prisoners chained two or three together. Their provision was put down to them through a hole in the floor of the room above; and those who served them there, often caught the fatal fever. At my first visit, I found the keeper, his assistant, and all the prisoners but one, sick of it; and heard that a few years before many prisoners had died of it – and the keeper and his wife in one night.[26]

There is no need to prolong this anatomy of abuses that Howard to his eternal honour exposed. Howard's data and descriptions make his verdict crystal clear. Gaols broke the law – most failed for instance to display, as was their obligation, the statutes regarding health of prisoners, the banning of garnish, gaming and the sale of spirits. Their administration was careless and often cruel. Ill-treated prisoners were herded into damp and dark cells, without proper ventilation, now too hot, now too cold; they lacked proper food, bedding, exercise or occupation. They were often cheated of their statutory or customary allowances – full-weight bread, for instance. Exorbitant mulcts and demands were imposed, like ward-dues or garnish, the levy on new inmates. Not least, as we have seen, convicts were often sick. What Howard called 'gaol fever' was rife, and frequently fatal to prisoners, keepers and staff alike, as his Launceston experience confirmed.[27]

State of the Prisons leaves no doubt about Howard's practical response to all this. He wished to ensure that magistrates and keepers be obliged to adhere to the letter of the law. He aimed to stamp out rackets and brutality. He wished to safeguard prisoners' physical health and well-being. He was anxious for their moral welfare. He wanted gaols efficient and accountable. He thus wrote as a lawyer, a utilitarian, a spiritual educator and a sanitarian. But he wrote, above all, from a broader perspective, one attentive, in a manner distinctive of the late Enlightenment, to environmental management, the moral economy of people and institutions, space and power.[28] To borrow John Bender's apt phrase, Howard was one of those involved in 'imagining the penitentiary',[29] creating a sanctuary of good management secured by a disciplinary regime.

What part in all this did the health of prisoners play? As will be evident by now, Howard was not moved exclusively by criteria of physical health, still less by a medical mission, targeted against typhus. He wanted good order. Wretched institutions were ruinous to health. 'There are prisons', he writes at the opening of the *State of the Prisons*:

> into which whoever looks will, at first sight of the people confined there, be convinced, that there is some great error in the management of them: their sallow meagre countenances declare, without words, that they are very miserable. Many who went in healthy, are in a few months changed to emaciated dejected objects. Some are seen pining under diseases, 'sick, and in prison'; expiring on the floors, in loathsome cells, of pestilential fevers, and the confluent smallpox; victims, I must not say to the cruelty, but I will say to the inattention, of sheriffs, and gentlemen in the commission of the peace.[30]

The prison sick-list was thus a warning signal, the alarming symptoms of a sick institution. In view of these priorities, it was never one of Howard's principal concerns to emplace the medical profession within gaols (though he did think that surgeons should be appointed). His axiom was that a properly-run gaol would necessarily be a salubrious gaol; and in that he followed contemporaries and comrades like Sir John Pringle, James Lind and James Cook, who were likewise arguing that the key to reducing scurvy and fevers amongst soldiers and sailors was not some medical miracle or machinery but rather maintaining, in the widest sense, a well-run army camp or barracks or a shipshape vessel.[31] There was a phrase in vogue in English lunatic asylums at this time that, for the alleviation of mental illness, management would do more than medicine.[32] I believe Howard and other institutional experts shared a similar sense of the paramountcy of order and regulation. It was undeniably to the fore in his thinking about gaols and lazarettos. He had already undertaken extensive rebuilding on his Bedfordshire estate, and was earnest for the moral supervision of his tenants and labourers. And an anecdote also tells us that, on marrying for the second time, he informed his wife 'that to prevent altercations about those little matters which he had observed to be the chief grounds of uneasiness in families, he should always decide'.[33] Blessed with boundless faith in the power of management, Howard advocated a number of directives for the comprehensive reform of gaols.[34] Buildings should be erected on airy sites near a stream or river; there must be adequate water and sanitation; overcrowding must cease; honest gaolers should be obtained, fees abolished and salaries substituted; prisoners' rations must be adequate – a vegetarian himself, he proposed a diet of bread, beans, soup, turnips and carrots; a surgeon or apothecary should be appointed to each gaol.

So how significant in Howard's imagination was gaol fever? The reformer, we must remember, was a philanthropist not a physician – though we are told that, when abroad, he chose to pass for a doctor, performing medical services – on one occasion delivering a baby aboard ship.[35] He had close medical friends, including Lind, and took considerable interest in medicine, thinking it advisable to apologize in the *State of the Prisons* lest he had trodden upon medical toes.[36] Hence, his views about gaol fever were doubtless the considered opinions of a medically well-informed layman. What he had to say is both frustrating and revealing.

As Howard saw it, there was an illness called gaol fever – sometimes he used terms like putrid fever or malignant fever – which was also rife in similar institutions like ships.[37] Howard regarded gaol fever as a self-evident diagnosis. He never saw the need to offer any more precise, more finely differentiated clinical description. He never felt required to assess its relations to other fevers and medical conditions. Throughout the *State of the Prisons*, he never referred to specific medical texts to anchor his views on fevers.[38] He never engaged in theoretical dispute regarding rival aetiological hypotheses, as for example the putative controversy between contagionists and miasmatists.[39] For Howard, gaol fever was a basic fact. It was the disorder of disordered institutions. More than once, he spelt out what precipitated it. It was due to a close atmosphere and want of ventilation. It followed from filth and overcrowding (a view confirmed by none other than the great Dr Haller, whom Howard met in Berne).[40] And it was encouraged by what we might call a personal, even psychological factor: morale. 'If it were asked', Howard reflected,

> what is the cause of gaol fever? it would in general be readily replied, 'the want of fresh air and cleanliness.' But as I have found in some

> prisons abroad, cells and dungeons as offensive and dirty as any I have observed in this country, where, however, this distemper was unknown, I am obliged to look out for some additional cause for its production. I am of the opinion, that the sudden change of diet and lodging so affects the spirits of new convicts, that the general causes of putrid fevers exert an immediate effect upon them. Hence it is common to see them sicken and die in a short time, with very little apparent illness. Convicts are generally stout robust young men, who have been accustomed to free diet, tolerable lodgings, and vigorous exercise. These are ironed, and thrust into close offensive dungeons, and there chained down, some of them, without straw or other bedding; in which they continue, in winter, sixteen or seventeen hours out of twenty-four, in utter inactivity, and immersed in the noxious effluvia of their own bodies. On this account, the gaol-distemper is always observed to reign more in our prisons during winter than summer; contract, I presume, to the nature of other putrid diseases. Their diet is at the same time low and scanty; they are generally without firing; and the powers of life soon become incapable of resisting so many causes of sickness and dispair.[41]

Thus if bad conditions in gaol formed the predisposing cause of the fever, there were exciting causes too. Howard believed that the trauma of incarceration, with its consequent lack of exercise and stimulus, so to speak reduced the powers of life or as we might say lowered resistance. (This notion that states of mind, fear for example, encouraged sickness, remained a commonplace, widely touted, for instance, during the nineteenth-century cholera outbreaks.)[42]

Howard saw gaol fever as a matter of moment. 'From my own observations in 1773, 1774, and 1775', he wrote, 'I was fully convinced that many more prisoners were destroyed by it, than were put to death by all the public executions in the kingdom'.[43] Its evil was multiplied because it could be spread beyond the gaol by released prisoners, if, for instance, they were impressed for military service. But from this it must not be inferred that Howard judged gaol fever contagious. His scepticism towards that possibility is evident from the fact that he snooped round gaols rather nonchalantly, convinced his sober habits, aided by Providence's protection, would safeguard him. 'To preserve myself from infection, in the hospitals and prisons I visit, next to the goodness and mercy of the Author of my being, temperance and cleanliness are my preservatives', he believed – albeit adding that 'I never enter an hospital or prison before breakfast, and in an offensive room I seldom draw my breath deeply'.[44]

From these and other hints, we may surmise that Howard was

inclined towards a *de facto* miasmatism when facing gaol fever and the maladies of prisons. Yet it would be wrong to leap to the conclusion that he was a doctrinaire miasmatist. He had no doubt, as he lengthily expounded in his *Account of the Principal Lazarettos in Europe*, that bubonic plague was contagious, smallpox too. Different disorders worked in different ways, and Howard in any case always emphasized the powerful role in disease susceptibility of individual constitutions and circumstances – how else could one explain the selective operations of sicknesses? 'Why, of a number of persons equally exposed to the infection of the small-pox, or of the gaol-fever, some will take it?', Howard inquired:

> Perhaps physicians themselves are not capable of explaining this sufficiently. It is, however, evident in general, that it must be owing to something in the state of the blood and the constitutions of such persons which renders them not easily susceptible of infection. – The rich are less liable to the plague than the poor, both because they are more careful to avoid infection, and have larger and more airy apartments, and because they are more cleanly and live on better food, with plenty of vegetables; and this, I suppose, is the reason why Protestants are less liable to this distemper than Catholics during their times of fasting; and, likewise, why the generality of Europeans are less liable to it than Greeks, and particularly Jews.[45]

In a series of publications, Margaret DeLacy has been developing the thesis that improvements in institutional hygiene and public health in the latter part of the eighteenth century arose from public-spirited reformers espousing contagionist positions and acting upon them.[46] Once identified as contagious, disease could be viewed, she believes, as a discrete entity subject to the laws of cause and effect, a tangible enemy that could be directly targeted. The doctrine of contagion encouraged active and positive responses, unlike, she implies, miasmatism which sanctioned a kind of fatalism (sickness was impalpable, elusive, just in the air). She may be right, though I am very sceptical about the affinity she postulates – after all, why shouldn't miasmatism galvanize action? All that was needed was a change of air![47] But her interpretation certainly doesn't hold good for Howard, who was endlessly preoccupied with combating the foul air and the 'closeness' of lock-ups.

DeLacy, however, is spot-on in one key respect: her delineation of the swell of prison reform in the eighteenth century, the mobilization of a movement. The heroic view of Howard as lone ranger – darkness reigned, then Howard rose and all was light – is no longer acceptable. Howard was one voice amongst a choir of critics of primitive prisons.

As early as 1701, the Society for the Propagation of Christian Knowledge sent a committee to visit Newgate, the Marshalsea and other prisons, finding them all deplorable.[48] In the 1720s Richard Mead, writing about plague, commented on the vitiated air of prisons; in February 1728, the Legislature appointed a Committee of the House of Commons to inquire into 'The State of the Gaols of this Kingdom', with Oglethorpe at its head.[49] In 1752, responding to the infamous 'black assizes' at Newgate, in which fifty people died of gaol fever, Stephen Hales and John Pringle developed mechanical ventilators to flood the gaols with air (Howard discovered a number of ventilators but few worked well).[50] In the last third of the century, numerous reformers debated the health of prisons in context of wider anxieties about epidemic disease and the salubrity of close-packed populations: hospitals, ships, hulks, camps, factories, workhouses, and urban slums: in these connections, the names of Haygarth, Heysham, Aikin, Perceval, Currie, Dobson, Lettsom, Lind and Pringle crop up again and again.[51] Specifically in prison reform, Jeremy Bentham (with his panopticon)[52] and Sir George Onesiphorus Paul (dedicated to the corrective rehabiliatory discipline of solitary confinement and redemptive labour) pioneered the penitentiary. Howard was thus one of many. Moreover, as DeLacy has rightly stressed, it would be wrong to assume too great a role for any individual *thinker*, that is for big ideas. As we know from the panopticon white elephant, grand designs often came to nothing. In 1779 an Act was passed empowering the erection of two penitentiary houses under the superintendence of three supervisors (19 Geo. III, c.74, sec. 5). Howard, Fothergill and Whatley, the treasurer of the Foundling Hospital, were appointed to undertake the experiment. They could not even agree about the site. Fothergill died in December 1780, Howard shortly afterwards sent in his resignation to Lord Bathurst, and the project ceased.

Not from philosophies, prison reform arose from practicalities, and it was generated from below, in the localities, amongst cabals of sheriffs, lords lieutenants and JPs. It arose out of local crisis, it proceeded piecemeal. Traditionally, as everyone knows, criminals were hanged, transported, whipped, fined or accorded mercy. Few had ended up serving long gaol sentences. Most of those in gaol had been debtors or those awaiting trial. Therefore gaols had been small and ramshackle and their makeshift nature had not mattered much. In the second half of the century, things changed. Population rose, crime rose; the prison population grew, especially when transportation of felons was drastically interrupted by American Independence – Howard himself referred to 1783 as the year 'when the prisons became crowded through the peace' and gaol sickness consequently worsened.[53] And the upshot of overcrowding was typhus – paralleling the worsening epidemics of the mushrooming towns. As DeLacy's study of Lancashire has demonstrated in resplendent detail, gaol overcrowding and disease left local magistrates with no option but to rebuild. And in the reconstruction process, magistrates incorporated a raft of design features – solitary confinement, prison uniforms, the abolition of the tap – meant to improve physical and spiritual well-being through the imposition of inescapable order.[54] Howard approved – and reforming magistrates often approved of Howard. But it was epidemics not Howard that got reform rolling.

Prisons, health, doctors and medicine: how, finally, were they connected in the eighteenth century? Gaols provided one locus amongst many for new attention to the sanitary problems of packed populations. They demanded a new optic and, to use Foucault's phrase, new disciplinary technologies.[55] In the real world, the rise of typhus required gaol reform, rather as the calamitous incidence of scurvy on trans-oceanic ships demanded a comprehensive new naval discipline.[56]

Necessity no less than philosophy propelled these reforms. A great debate, launched by Oliver MacDonagh, has raged amongst nineteenth-century historians regarding the explanation of the rise of the Victorian administrative state: was it due to Benthamism or ineluctable necessity?[57] The pragmatists have probably had the better of the argument. The same, I suggest, applies before 1800. Typhus proved the best prison reformer.

And when prison reform came, it was not led by physicians, still less by the medical profession and its colleges and coteries. It focused not on a regime of preventive and curative medicine, but the construction of perfectly regulated environments. There may well be scope for violently differing readings of the prison medical service, as it developed in the nineteenth century: the prisoner's friend, or the lackey of authority?[58] But at the death of Howard in 1790, the idea of a prison medical service had not even been broached.[59] Medicine was not ready for such responsibilities. In England at least, it was only in the nineteenth century that medicine formed itself into a professional lobby, a caucus, a fifth, sixth or seventh estate, the natural proxy of suffering humanity.[60]

Notes

1. Quoted in John Gibson, 'John Howard and the Gaol-fever', *History of Medicine*, vii (1976), 49–54, 50.
2. For the apotheosis of Howard, see for instance [anon.], *The Vindication*

of Fame. An Ode in Honour of John Howard (London, 1786); [anon.], *The Protection of Providence: An Ode. Sacred to the Fame of Mr Howard* (London: T. Cadell and G. Nicoll, 1787); [Samuel Jackson Pratt], *The Triumph of Benevolence; Occasioned by the National Design of Erecting a Monument to John Howard, Esq* (Dublin: Byrne, 1786).

3. William Hepworth Dixon, *John Howard and the Prison World of Europe*, 2nd edn (London: Jackson and Walford, 1850), 1.
4. The Rt Hon. Merlyn Rees, 'Opening Statement', in John C. Freeman (ed.), *Prisons Past and Future* (London: Heinemann, 1978), 1.
5. A good account of these progressive and largely Dissenting circles is James Johnston Abraham, *Lettsom. His Life, Times, Friends and Descendants* (London: William Heinemann, 1933); see also R. Hingston Fox, *Dr John Fothergill and His Friends: Chapters in Eighteenth Century Life* (London: Macmillan & Co., 1919). The views of Lind etc. are discussed in John Gibson, 'John Howard and the Gaol-fever', *History of Medicine*, vii (1976), 49–54, 52f.; and John E. Ransom, 'John Howard on Communicable Diseases', *Bulletin of the Institute of the History of Medicine*, v (1937), 131–47; *idem*, 'John Howard on Quarantine', *Bulletin of the Institute of the History of Medicine*, vi (1938), 111–16, who notes the tendency of Lind to blame typhus outbreaks on board ship on sailors impressed from gaols. For these groups see ch. 3, 'Gaol Fever', in R. Evans, *The Fabrication of Virtue: English Prison Architecture 1750–1840* (Cambridge: Cambridge University Press, 1982).
6. L. Baumgartner, 'John Howard and the Public Health Movement', *Bulletin of the Institute of the History of Medicine*, v (1937), 489–508, 489.
7. For Howard as proto-sanitarian, see L. Baumgartner, 'John Howard and the Public Health Movement', *Bulletin of the Institute of the History of Medicine*, v (1937), 489–508; William A. Guy, *John Howard's Winter Journey* (London: De La Rue, 1882); *idem, 1773; or John Howard, Sheriff of Bedford* (London: Henry Renshaw, 1873); *idem*, 'John Howard as a Statist', *Journal of the Statistical Society*, xxxvi (1873), 1–18; *idem*, 'John Howard's True Place in History. A Supplement to the Paper Entitled 'John Howard as a Statist', *Journal of the Statistical Society*, xxxviii (1875), 430–7. Guy was attempting to appropriate Howard as an early hero of the public health movement. Guy said he preferred not to look upon Howard as a philanthropist. See also Benjamin Ward Richardson, 'John Howard, LLD, F.R.S.', in *Disciples of Aesculapius*, 2 vols (London: Hutchinson and Co., 1900), vol. ii, 751–68. For the earlier vision of Howard the Christian martyr see [anon.], *Christian Biography, Containing the Lives of Rich. Baxter, Mrs M. Baxter, J. Howard, Claudius Buchanan, Viscountess Glenorchy* (London: Religious Tract Society, 1832–3).
8. This story was, it seems, more than mere gossip. It was believed by many of Howard's friends and admirers, including John Coakley Lettsom.

9. Thomas Carlyle, *Collected Works. Latter-day Pamphlets* (London: Chapman and Hall, 1850), vol. xix, 75–80; see also [William A. Guy], 'Thomas Carlyle and John Howard', *Fraser's Magazine*, xli (1850), 400–10.
10. Rod Morgan, 'Divine Philanthropy: John Howard Reconsidered', *History*, lxii (1977), 388–410 is rather splenetic in its iconoclasm. For broader attempts to abandon the sentimental vision of the prisoner's friend and stress reform as an intensification of the disciplinary system, see Michael Ignatieff, *A Just Measure of Pain: The Penitentiary in the Industrial Revolution, 1750–1850* (London: Macmillan, 1978); M. Foucault, *Discipline and Punish: The Birth of the Prison* (Harmondsworth: Penguin, 1979); Dario Melossi and Massimo Pavarini, *The Prison and the Factory* (London: Macmillan, 1981).
11. For basic biographical information, the *Dictionary of National Biography* article remains valuable. The book-length biographies add rather little. But see John Aikin, *A View of the Character and Public Services of the Late John Howard* (London: J. Johnson, 1792). Howard deserves a new scholarly study.
12. Eric Stockdale, 'John Howard and Bedford Prison', in John C. Freeman (ed.), *Prisons Past and Future* (London: Heinemann, 1978), 15–24. For the role of Howard and Samuel Whitbread in reforming Bedford institutions, see Bernard Cashman, *Private Charity and the Public Purse. The Development of Bedford General Hospital 1794–1988* (Bedford: North Bedfordshire Health Authority, 1988); *idem, A Proper House: Bedford Lunatic Asylum (1812–1860)* (Bedford: North Bedfordshire Health Authority, 1992).
13. John Howard, *The State of the Prisons*, 3rd edn (Warrington and London: T Cadell, 1784), 2: 'Upon this subject I was examined in the House of Commons in March 1774: when I had the honour of their thanks. Soon after that, Mr. Popham, member for Taunton, repeated the humane attempt which had miscarried a few years before; and brought in a bill for the relief of prisoners who should be acquired – respecting their fees; and another bill for preserving the health of prisoners, and preventing the gaol-distemper. They both passed, that sessions: these two acts I had printed in a different character, and sent them to the keeper of every county gaol in England. By those acts, the tear was wiped from many an eye; and the legislature had for them the blessing of many that were ready to perish.' The Act is as follows: A.D. 1774. Anno 14° Georgii III, c.57,58,59. 697–699 C A P. LIX – 'An Act for preserving the Health of Prisoners in Gaol, and preventing the Gaol Distemper': 'WHEREAS the malignant Fever, that is commonly called *The Gaol Distemper*, is found to be owing to a want of Cleanliness and fresh Air in the several Gaols in *England* and *Wales*, and the fatal Consequences of that Disorder, of which there has been of late too much Experience, might be prevented if Justices of the Peace were duly authorized to provide such Accommodations in Gaols

as may be necessary to answer this salutary Purpose: May it therefore please Your Majesty that it may be enacted; and be it enacted by the King's Most Excellent Majesty, by and with the Advice and Consent of the Lords Spiritual and Temporal, and Commons, in this present Parliament assembled, and by the Authority of the same, That the several Justices of the Peace in that Part of *Great Britain* called *England* and *Wales*, within their several Jurisdictions, in their Quarter-Sessions assembled, are hereby authorised and required to order the Walls and Ceilings of the several Cells and Wards, both of the Debtors and the Felons, and also of any other Rooms used by the Prisoners in their respective Gaols and Prisons where Felons are usually confined, to be seraged and white-washed. Once in the Year at least; to be regularly washed and kept clean, and constantly supplied with fresh Air by means of Hand Ventilators, or other wise; to order Two Rooms in each Gaol or Prison, one for the Men and the other for the Women, to be set apart for the Sick Prisoners, directing them to be removed into such Rooms as soon as they shall be seized with an Disorder, and kept separate from those who shall be in Health; to order a Warm and Cold Bath, or commodious Bathing Tubs, according to the Condition in which they shall be at the Time, before they are suffered to go out of such Gaols or Prisons upon any Occasion whatever; to order this Act to be painted in large and legible Characters upon a Board, and hung up in form conspicuous Part of each of the said Gaols and Prisons; and to appoint an experienced Surgeon or Apothecary, at a stated Salary, to attend each Gaol or Prison respectively, who shall and he is hereby directed to report to the said Justices by whom he is appointed, at each Quarter-Sessions, a State of the Health of the Prisoners, under his Care of Superintendence.'

14. Compare the Madhouses Act of the same year, which required magistrates to license and empowered them to inspect private lunatic asylums. See William Llewellyn Parry-Jones, *The Trade in Lunacy: A Study of Private Madhouses in England in the Eighteenth and Nineteenth Centuries* (London: Routledge & Kegan Paul, 1971).
15. L. Baumgartner, 'John Howard (1726–1790), Hospital and Prison Reformer: A Bibliography', *Bulletin of the History of Medicine*, vii (1939), 595–626. In this paper I shall be wholly concerned with Howard's work on prisons; I shall not examine his work on lazarettos.
16. William H. Dixon, *John Howard and the Prison World of Europe*, 2nd edn (London: Jackson and Walford, 1850), 228.
17. Michael Ignatieff, *A Just Measure of Pain: The Penitentiary in the Industrial Revolution, 1750–1850* (London: Macmillan, 1978); M. Foucault, *Discipline and Punish: The Birth of the Prison* (Harmondsworth: Penguin, 1979).
18. On Bentham see Janet Semple, 'Bentham's Utilitarianism and the Provision of Medical Care', in Dorothy Porter and Roy Porter (editors), *Doctors, Politics and Society: Historical Essays* (Amsterdam:

Rodopi, 1993), 30–46.

19. Alongside the work of Foucault and Ignatieff already mentioned, Margaret DeLacy, *Prison Reform in Lancashire, 1700–1850* (Manchester: Chetham Society, 1986) and R. Evans, *The Fabrication of Virtue: English Prison Architecture 1750–1840* (Cambridge: Cambridge University Press, 1982) are exceptionally valuable. See also J. A. Sharpe, *Crime in Early Modern England 1550–1750* (London: Longman, 1984); J. M. Beattie, *Crime and the Courts in England, 1660–1800* (Oxford: Oxford University Press, 1986); Joanna Innes, 'The King's Bench Prison in the Later Eighteenth Century: Law, Authority and Order in a London Debtor's Prison', in John Brewer and John Styles (eds), *An Ungovernable People: The English and their Law in the Seventeenth and Eighteenth Centuries* (London: Hutchinson, 1980), 250–98; *idem*, 'Prisons for the Poor: English Bridewells, 1555–1640', in F. Snyder and D. Hay (eds), *Labour, Law and Crime: An Historical Perspective* (London: Tavistock, 1987), 42–122; *idem*, 'Politics and Morals: The Reformation of Manners Movement in Later Eighteenth-Century England', in Eckhart Hellmuth (ed.), *The Transformation of Political Culture* (London: Oxford University Press, 1990), 57–118; J. Innes and J. Styles, 'The Crime Wave: Recent Writing on Crime and Criminal Justice in Eighteenth Century England', *Journal of British Studies*, xxv (1986), 380–435.

20. R. Evans, *The Fabrication of Virtue: English Prison Architecture 1750–1840* (Cambridge: Cambridge University Press, 1982) is the major study to which I am deeply indebted – for Blackburn see 170f.; F. G. Neild, 'James Neild and Prison Reform', *Journal of the Royal Society of Medicine*, lxxiv (1981), 834–40 – Neild was a Quaker jeweller from London and secretary of the Society for the Relief and Discharge of Persons Imprisoned for Small Debts. He made it his business, at the request of John Coakley Lettsom, to tread in Howard's footsteps and visit most of the English gaols; Brian Hill, 'Irons in the Fire: John Mason Good, MD (1764–1827)', *The Practitioner*, cxcii (1964), 697–700: a versatile London physician, in 1795 J.M. Good, who was the physician at Coldbath Fields Prison, responded to a request from the Medical Society of London by publishing *A Dissertation on the Diseases of Prisons and Workhouses*, in which he argued that 'the greater number of all disorders in prisons and workhouses proceeded from inattention to cloathing and cleanliness'. He suggested Howardian reforms. Good had long boasted of his friendship with Howard as a source of 'high benefit and advantage'. See the discussion in Joe Sim, *The Prison Medical Service in England 1774–1989* (Milton Keynes: Open University Press, 1990), 12. For the general subject, see Christine Stevenson, 'Medicine and Architecture', in W. F. Bynum and Roy Porter (eds), *Companion Encyclopedia of the History of Medicine* (London: Routledge, 1993), vol. ii, 1495–1519.

21. Pieter Spierenburg, *The Prison Experience: Disciplinary Institutions and Their Inmates in Early Modern Europe* (New Brunswick/London: Rutgers University Press, 1991); Howard, *State of the Prisons* (London: Dent, 1928), 46f.
22. Howard, *State of the Prisons* (Warrington and London: T Cadell, 1777), 329.
23. Howard, *State of the Prisons*, 358.
24. Howard, *State of the Prisons*, 362–3.
25. Howard, *State of the Prisons*, 382–3.
26. Howard, *State of the Prisons*, 391.
27. Howard, *State of the Prisons*, 469.
28. Howard, *State of the Prisons*, 470–2.
29. For Enlightenment attempts to diagnose disease and improve health through examination of man's relationship to his environment, natural and artificial, see L. J. Jordanova, 'Earth Science and Environmental Medicine: The Synthesis of the Late Enlightenment', in L. J. Jordanova and Roy Porter (eds), *Images of the Earth: Essays in the History of the Environmental Sciences* (Chalfont St Giles: British Society for the History of Science Monographs, 1979), 119–46; Clarence J. Glacken, *Traces on the Rhodian Shore* (Berkeley: University of California Press, 1967); James C. Riley, 'The Medicine of the Environment in Eighteenth-Century Germany', *Clio Medica*, xviii (1983), 167–78; *idem, The Eighteenth Century Campaign to Avoid Disease* (Basingstoke: Macmillan, 1987). For the parallel with the internal economy of the asylum, see Christine Stevenson, 'Madness and the Picturesque in the Kingdom of Denmark', in W. F. Bynum, Roy Porter & M. Shepherd (eds), *The Anatomy of Madness: Essays in the History of Psychiatry*, vol. 3 (London: Tavistock Publications, 1987), 13–47; and Roy Porter, *Mind Forg'd Manacles: Madness and Psychiatry in England from Restoration to Regency* (London, Athlone Press, 1987; paperback edition, Penguin, 1990); Christopher Paul Philo, 'The Space Reserved for Insanity: Studies in the Historical Geography of the Mad-Business in England and Wales' (University of Cambridge, Ph.D. thesis, 1992); T. A. Markus (ed.), *Order in Space and Society* (Edinburgh: Mainstream Publishing Co., 1982).
30. Howard, *State of the Prisons*, 4.
31. There is a fine conceptual and empirical discussion in C. J. Lawrence, 'Disciplining Disease: Scurvy, the Navy, and Imperial Expansion 1750–1825', in D. Miller and P. Reill (eds), *Visions of Empire* (Cambridge: Cambridge University Press, forthcoming). For the exemplary case of Blyth, see Greg Dening, *Mr Bligh's Bad Language* (Cambridge: Cambridge University Press, 1992).
32. Roy Porter, 'Was there a Moral Therapy in Eighteenth Century Psychiatry?', *Lychnos* (1981–2), 12–26.
33. James Baldwin Brown, *Memoirs of the Public and Private Life of John Howard* (London: Rest Fenner, 1818), 55.

34. Howard, *State of the Prisons*, 469.
35. William H. Dixon, *John Howard and the Prison World of Europe*, 2nd edn (London: Jackson and Walford, 1850), 334; [anon.], *Anecdotes of the Life and Character of J H. Written by a Gentleman, whose Acquaintance with that Celebrated Philanthropist gave him the most Favourable Opportunity of Learning Particulars not Generally Known* (London: Hookham etc., 1790), 26.
36. Howard, *State of the Prisons*, 467. At the end of *State of Prisons*, Howard adds a chapter which he entitles 'Remarks on the Gaol Fever'. He says: 'I shall take the liberty here to subjoin a few additional remarks on the gaol fever; in which, if I shall appear to have invaded the province of the gentlemen of the faculty, I hope to be pardoned, from the consideration that my experience in this matter, may in some respect supply my want of other means of knowledge'.
37. Gaol fever is now generally recognized as typhus. For typhus see Anne Hardy, 'Typhus in the Victorian City', *Medical History*, xxxii (1988), 401–25; Guenter Risse, 'Typhus' Fever in Eighteenth-century Hospitals: New Approaches to Medical Treatment', *Bulletin of the History of Medicine*, lix (1985), 176–95; D. C. Smith, 'Medical Science, Medical Practice, and the Emerging Concept of Typhus in Mid-Eighteenth-Century Britain', in W. F. Bynum and V. Nutton (eds), *Theories of Fever from Antiquity to the Enlightenment* (London: Medical History Supplement no. 1, London, Wellcome Institute for the History of Medicine, 1981), 121–34 – the whole volume is valuable; H. Zinsser, *Rats, Lice and History* (Boston, Mass.: Atlantic Monthly Press, Little, Brown & Co., 1935). It was widely thought at the time that gaol fever resulted from overcrowding. Putrid fevers, wrote John Haygarth, 'are generated by a great number of persons crowded together in the same room as in a ship, jail, etc': John Haygarth, *A Letter to Dr Percival on the Prevention of Infectious Fevers* (Bath: Cruttwell, 1801), 45.
38. He might have cited, because he probably had read, some of the following: John Huxham, *Observations On The Air And Epidemic Diseases* (London: J. Hinton, 1759); *idem*, *An Essay On Fevers* (London: J. Hinton, 1769); John Pringle, *Observations on the Nature and Cure of Hospital and Jayl Fevers* (London: Millar and Wilson, 1750).
39. Historians of medicine have made much of the so-called struggle between miasmatists and contagionists. It is disputable whether that battle was real or is simply a convenient historians' construct. See Margaret Pelling, 'Contagion/Germ Theory/Specificity', in W. F. Bynum and Roy Porter (eds), *Routledge Companion Encyclopaedia to the History of Medicine* (London: Routledge, 1993), 309–34; *idem*, *Cholera, Fever and English Medicine 1825–1865* (Oxford: Oxford University Press, 1978); O. Temkin, 'An Historical Analysis of the Concept of Infection', in *The Double Face of Janus and Other Essays in the History of Medicine* (Baltimore & London: Johns Hopkins University Press,

1977), 456–71; *idem*, 'The Scientific Approach to Disease; Specific Entity and Individual Sickness', in A. L. Caplan, H. T. Engelhardt, Jr. and J. J. McCartney (eds), *Concepts of Health and Disease: Interdisciplinary Perspectives* (Reading, Mass.: Addison-Wesley Publishing Co., 1981), 247–63; R. Cooter, 'Anticontagionism and History's Medical Record', in P. Wright and A. Treacher (eds), *The Problem of Medical Knowledge* (Edinburgh: Edinburgh University Press, 1982), 87–108; and, the best recent discussion, C. Hamlin, 'Predisposing Causes and Public Health in Early Nineteenth Century Medical Thought', *Social History of Medicine*, v (1992), 43–70.

40. William H. Dixon, *John Howard and the Prison World of Europe*, 2nd edn (London: Jackson and Walford, 1850), 200.
41. Howard, *State of the Prisons*, 467.
42. M. Durey, *The Return of the Plague: British Society and the Cholera 1831–2* (Dublin: Gill & Macmillan, 1979); R. J. Morris, 'Religion and Medicine: The Cholera Pamphlets of Oxford 1832, 1849 and 1854', *Medical History*, xix (1975), 256–70; *idem*, *Cholera, 1832: The Social Response to an Epidemic* (London: Croom Helm, 1976).
43. Howard, *State of the Prisons*, 8–9.
44. Howard, *An Account of the Principal Lazarettos in Europe* (Warrington and London: T Cadell, 1789), 232. The relations between personal and environmental cleanliness are well explored in Alain Corbin, *The Foul and the Fragrant: Order and the French Social Imagination* (Cambridge, Mass.: Harvard University Press, 1986) and Virginia S. Smith, 'Cleanliness: the Development of an Idea and Practice in Britain 1770–1850' (University of London, Ph.D. thesis, 1985); *idem*, 'The Physiology of Air: Eighteenth-Century Fever Therapy in the Advice Literature', *Bulletin of the Society for the Social History of Medicine*, xxxv (1984), 21–3.
45. Howard, *An Account of the Principal Lazarettos in Europe* (Warrington and London: T Cadell, 1789), 25.
46. Margaret DeLacy, *Prison Reform in Lancashire, 1700–1850* (Manchester: Chetham Society, 1986); *idem*, 'The Conceptualization of Influenza in Eighteenth-century Britain: Specificity and Contagion', *Bulletin of the History of Medicine*, lxvii (1993), 74–118; *idem*, 'Puerperal Fever in Eighteenth-Century Britain', *Bulletin of the History of Medicine*, lxiii (1989), 521–56. DeLacy thereby disputes the commonplace that it was miasmatism or anti-contagionism that bred public health activism.
47. Instances where miasmatist doctrines clearly spurred action are offered in James C. Riley, *The Eighteenth Century Campaign to Avoid Disease* (Basingstoke: Macmillan, 1987), and Roy Porter, 'Cleaning Up The Great Wen: Public Health in Eighteenth Century London', in W. F. Bynum and Roy Porter (eds), *Living and Dying in London* (*Medical History* supplement 11, London: Wellcome Institute for the History of Medicine, 1991), 61–75. Many historians have precisely believed that

adherence to miasmatism spurred public health activism.

48. William A. Guy, 'John Howard's True Place in History. A Supplement to the Paper Entitled 'John Howard as a Statist'', *Journal of the Statistical Society*, xxxviii (1875), 430–7, 435.
49. An intelligent reading of Oglethorpe is offered in John Bender, *Imagining the Penitentiary. Fiction and the Architecture of Mind in Eighteenth Century England* (Chicago: University of Chicago Press, 1987), 17; see also Donna T. Andrew, *Philanthropy and Police: London Charity in the Eighteenth Century* (Princeton, N. J.: Princeton University Press, 1989). On 25 February, 1728, the Legislature appointed a Committee of the House of Commons to inquire into 'The State of the Gaols of this Kingdom', and report to it thereon.
50. Howard, *State of the Prisons*, 347.
51. See above all Ulrich Tröhler, 'Quantification in British Medicine and Surgery 1750–1830; with Special Reference to its Introduction into Therapeutics' (Ph.D. thesis, University of London, 1978); *idem*, 'To Improve the Evidence of Medicine: Arithmetic Observation in Clinical Medicine in the Eighteenth and Early Nineteenth Centuries', *History and Philosophy of Life Sciences*, x (1988), 31–40; Simon Schaffer, 'Measuring Virtue: Eudiometry, Enlightenment and Pneumatic Medicine', in Andrew Cunningham and Roger French (eds), *The Medical Enlightenment of the Eighteenth Century* (Cambridge: Cambridge University Press, 1990), 281–318; R. Kilpatrick, '"Living in the Light": Dispensaries, Philanthropy and Medical Reform in Late-eighteenth Century London', in *ibid.*, 254–80, and Francis M. Lobo, 'John Haygarth, Smallpox and Religious Dissent in Eighteenth-Century England', in *ibid.*, 217–53; John Pickstone, 'Ferriar's Fever to Kay's Cholera: Disease and Social Structure in Cottonopolis', *History of Science*, xxii (1984), 401–19.
52. Janet Semple, 'Bentham's Utilitarianism and the Provision of Medical Care', in Dorothy Porter and Roy Porter (eds), *Doctors, Politics and Society: Historical Essays* (Amsterdam: Rodopi, 1993), 30–46.
53. Howard, *State of the Prisons*, 3rd edn (Warrington and London: T Cadell, 1784), 468.
54. Far the best account is contained in Margaret DeLacy, *Prison Reform in Lancashire, 1700–1850* (Manchester: Chetham Society, 1986); see especially 76 f.
55. See Colin Jones and Roy Porter (eds), *Reassessing Foucault: Power, Medicine and the Body*, (London: Routledge, 1994), especially Felix Driver, 'Bodies in Space: Foucault's Account of Disciplinary Power', 113–31. See also Dorinda Outram, *The Body and the French Revolution: Sex, Class and Political Culture* (New Haven, Conn.: Yale University Press, 1989). For another, and rather more sympathetic, assessment, see Bryan S. Turner, *The Body and Society: Explorations in Social Theory* (Oxford: Basil Blackwell, 1984); 'The Practices of Rationality: Michel Foucault, Medical History and Sociological Theory', in R. Fardon (ed.),

Power and Knowledge: Anthropological and Sociological Approaches (Edinburgh: Scottish Academic Press, 1985), 193–213; and *Medical Power and Social Knowledge* (Beverly Hills, Calif.: Sage, 1987).

56. See C. J. Lawrence's admirably penetrating 'Disciplining Disease: Scurvy, the Navy, and Imperial Expansion 1750–1825', in D. Miller and P. Reill (eds), *Visions of Empire* (Cambridge: Cambridge University Press, forthcoming). Evans has emphasized that reformers often invoked Howard's name to sanction reforms that necessity required: R. Evans, *The Fabrication of Virtue: English Prison Architecture 1750–1840* (Cambridge: Cambridge University Press, 1982), 139.
57. O. MacDonagh, *Early Victorian Government* (London: Weidenfeld and Nicolson, 1977); *idem*, 'The Nineteenth Century Revolution in Government: A Reappraisal', *Historical Journal*, i (1958), 52–67; G. Kitson Clark, 'Statesmen in Disguise: Reflections on the History of the Neutrality of the Civil Service', *Historical Journal*, ii (1959), 19–39; J. Bartlett Brebner, 'Laissez-faire and State Intervention in Nineteenth-Century Britain', *Journal of Economic History*, viii (1948), Supp., 59–73; Henry Parris, 'The Nineteenth-Century Revolution in Government: A Reappraisal Reappraised', *Historical Journal*, iii (1960), 17–37; Robert M. Gutchen, 'Local Improvements and Centralization in Nineteenth Century England', *Historical Journal*, iv (1961), 85–96; Jenifer Hart, 'Nineteenth Century Social Reform: A Tory Interpretation of History', *Past and Present*, xxxi (July 1965), 39–61; L. J. Hume, 'Jeremy Bentham and the Nineteenth Century Revolution in Government', *Historical Journal*, x (1967), 361–75; William C. Lubenow, *The Politics of Government Growth: Early Victorian Attitude Toward State Intervention 1833–1848* (Newton Abbot: David and Charles, 1971); S. E. Finer, 'The Transmission of Benthamite Ideas 1820–50', in Gillian Sutherland (ed.), *Studies in the Growth of Nineteenth Century Government* (London: Routledge and Kegan Paul, 1972), 11–32; David Roberts, 'Jeremy Bentham and the Victorian Administrative State', *Victorian Studies*, ii (1959), 193–210; *idem*, *Paternalism in Early Victorian England* (New Brunswick, N.J.: Rutgers University Press, 1979).
58. See the excellent history by Joe Sim: *The Prison Medical Service in England 1774–1989* (Milton Keynes: Open University Press, 1990).
59. Sim, *The Prison Medical Service.*
60. For discussion of the power politics of medicine in the nineteenth century, see Dorothy Porter and Roy Porter (eds), *Doctors, Politics and Society: Historical Essays* (Amsterdam: Rodopi, 1993), especially the Introduction.

Commentary

Bynum Why among a great many reformers has Howard been singled out for praise and recognition?

Porter In many other fields people like to adopt founder figures and invest them with status and hagiography. But the real and tangible reason is absolutely plain: two great books, and none of the other writers on prison reform did more than produce articles and bits and pieces in the periodical press. And most of the real prison reform that was going on in the counties left almost nothing on paper, whereas in Howard we have the big prison book in the library which could be assimilated into the whole great tradition of reformism. I think it is the books that make the difference: they are wonderful books as Dr Creese was saying earlier.

Porter (in answer to a question) Howard never left on paper any reflection upon the psychology or motivation of prisoners. He was really interested in environmental management, though not quite in a Skinnerian way. Howard thought that if you provide the right sort of institution then that solves the problem, or at least that is the way to solve the problem: he was not interested in criminology so far as I am aware.

Porter (in response to a question by Smith) Howard not being a medical man was relatively uninterested in the causes of diseases. That was not his prime concern: he was interested in their incidence as an index of a bad institution and he thought that institutions should be made good. He was not in a general sense interested in the aetiology of fevers or things like that: he was interested primarily in managing institutions, and questions of the causes of disease were secondary for him.

2

Medical Treatment and Prisoners' Health in Stafford Gaol during the Eighteenth Century

Anthony John Standley

An aspect of imprisonment during the eighteenth century, not always appreciated, is that the Keeper of the County Gaol was not a paid official. His was an office of profit whereby he obtained such monetary reward as he could from the persons in his charge. Indeed the Gaoler may well have had another occupation and would probably have benefited from the supply of beer to the prisoners. The Gaoler was required to pay an annual rent for the Gaol building. He may have purchased his situation but just how he came by office in Staffordshire at that time is not at all clear. In law the Gaoler was the servant of the Sheriff, but as the Sheriff held office for only a period of one year continuity in the supervision of the Gaoler was minimal. In respect of Houses of Correction, which after all was another form of imprisonment where the culprit was sent to work, then the Master could receive wages. At times the same person held both offices, Keeper of the Gaol and Master of the House of Correction, but not during the major part of the time under consideration. That situation expressed, it may be possible to view the period, as far as is possible given the limited specific information at hand, with some modest understanding of the Gaoler's situation, without suggesting that it should now meet with our approval.

The principal function of a County Gaol in the earlier part of the eighteenth century was to ensure that those persons committed to the custody of the Gaoler were kept secure until discharged by process of law. The largest group of prisoners was possibly those held awaiting trial (this would include those persons prisoner as a consequence of not being able to provide surety or security for their attendance at Court) and due to appear either at the Assizes presided over by Judges who would visit the County in the course of a circuit twice during the year, about Lent and late Summer, or at the County Quarter Sessions of the Peace, which were held by the Justices of the Peace of the County at Michaelmas, Epiphany, Easter and Midsummer. Additionally there would be those persons unable to give security for the performance of an order of the Court and held in custody until the matter was resolved. Another and at times substantial group included those confined in consequence of debt and for whom throughout the period there was a succession of Acts of Parliament to help secure their release. Imprisonment as a punitive measure in the earlier part of the century, while possible, was not nearly as common then as today, but increased towards the end of the period. Dependent upon the seriousness of the offence a whipping or a fine would more likely have been imposed, while if a custodial period as a reformative measure was considered necessary there existed the Houses of Correction in which those persons who were committed there could be put to employment. That establishment was, however, originally intended for idle vagrants and the offences that prisoners had committed did not always qualify them to be sent there. For more serious offenders the death penalty loomed or, mitigating the severity of this, there was transportation, at the beginning of the century to the Americas, at the end of it to Australia.

At the beginning of the period if any medical treatment was required the individual prisoner would be expected to make provision for it. This would not have been difficult, providing the prisoner had sufficient means, inasmuch as access to prisoners by members of the public was far easier then. Those prisoners who were – in terms of security – at risk, would have been personally secured by chains. The attendance of an Apothecary or a Surgeon would have posed no problem.

Where a woman was delivered of a child in the Gaol or House of Correction then a Midwife could attend.[1] Maintaining a child born to a parent that died in the Gaol could also lead to expense for the Gaoler who would hope to reclaim this from the County (as happened when Ann Davenhill was burnt for poisoning her husband in 1703).[2] Where a prisoner died in the Gaol and was without friends or family to claim the body, then the County generally repaid the Gaoler the costs of burial.[3]

There was originally no provision in law to feed prisoners whilst in prison, merely a Christian duty not to let them die from starvation. Since food is vital for health, its provision became a responsibility of the County and a sum of money was levied on the ratepayers to this end, the Gaoler receiving an annual sum to provide for the felons (in 1706 it was twenty pounds per year made in two payments at Michaelmas and LadyDay).[4] From the very end of the seventeenth century debtor prisoners were also given an allowance for bread following a petition made by them to the County Justices in which they claimed that they were trying to survive on the allowance given the felons.[5] Prisoners in the House of Correction were required to work for their keep, but an allowance was later extended to them also.[6]

With odd exceptions the Gaols of the country served the local community, in the present case that of the County of Stafford. It had earlier been considered advisable that Gaols should be made in populous places, where the charity of the locals could relieve those destitute of means.[7] Charity boxes were a feature at Gaols, where passers-by could make donations. Legacies for the benefit of poor prisoners were not unknown, though by no means frequent.[8]

There is little direct information about the condition of the Gaol at the beginning of the period or the size or number of the chambers. Individual cells were then a thing of the future. There is also a slight complication since in the past Stafford had had two Gaols, one serving the County, one the Borough. Towards the end of the first Queen Elizabeth's reign there appears, however, to have been one Gaol only and it was used by the County, and for this the County paid rent, a situation that satisfied the Borough of Stafford because while the County had a Gaol at Stafford it more or less guaranteed that the Assizes and Quarter Sessions would also be held at Stafford, bringing business to the advantage of the Townsmen. By the beginning of the eighteenth century, however, the County had its own Gaol although it is not so clear if, or for how long, the Borough continued with a Gaol of its own.[9]

This latest County Gaol, built in 1621, had been enlarged circa 1687, having then been described as 'much out of repair and by reason of the shortness and small compass of rooms become noisome and unwholesome to the prisoners, whereby many of them are lately dead and more likely and in danger of dying'. The work cost some £200 and further repairs were carried out a year or two afterwards. Such alterations and repairs do not tell us much about the situation but we can at least see that at times something was done by the Justices of the County – that unpaid workforce of yesteryear – and repairs are not an infrequent item on the County expenditure. Oversight of the work was normally given to selected persons, the Clerk of the Peace, the County Treasurer and perhaps one or two of the Justices, so that it would be carried out to the best advantage of the County.[10]

In 1714 the County raised more money to alter the Gaol and build a new House of Correction, the roof to be covered with lead, the overall cost being some £500.[11]

1727 brought the appointment by the County Justices of the Reverend William Corne, Curate of St Mary's, Stafford, to preach and read prayers to the poor prisoners in the Gaol and a room at the Gaol was fitted up for this purpose. The Reverend Corne's duties were to read prayers every Wednesday, Friday, Sunday and Holy-day and to give a sermon once a month or more. He was also to attend the condemned felons. The term 'poor prisoners' quite often, but not always, denotes the debtors and I draw the conclusion that it was for their benefit and not that of the felons that this arrangement was made, since if the clergyman was also dealing with the other prisoners there would not be need to specify attending the condemned felons, unless that requirement was intended to include attendance at the actual execution, in those days carried out in public and at some distance from the Gaol. It is vague. For this work Corne was to receive £10 per year.[12]

The first instance of payment being made to a medical man now occurs. In 1728 Francis Lee, Surgeon, was to be paid £2 for bleeding and purging 'the late transports before they were conveyed to Liverpool'. A few years before this date a revised policy for taking prisoners out of the country had been introduced. Whereas before those sentenced to transportation had been required to leave the country of their own accord, a condition not always complied with, they were now to be taken by a contractor. Since they were confined until this was done it appears to have become a County responsibility – perhaps limitedly – to look after their health while in the Gaol and details of expenditure subsequently occur.[13]

In 1729 the Gaoler was reimbursed for meat and necessary provisions found by him for several sick prisoners, while an Apothecary, Mr Abnett, received £2–4s–8d.[14] Later that year surgery was again carried out on 'transports' by Francis Lee; again he received £2.[15]

During the first half of 1729/30 a further £4–14s–2d was paid for expenditure on 25 prisoners who had been sick, 7 of whom had died. Authority for their treatment had been given by John Wedgewood and John Jarvis, two of the Justices of the Peace.[16] In the very earliest reference to expenditure the details of the treatment given, if originally submitted, do not survive, but for a nine-month period of 1729/30 the Apothecary's bill submitted to the Justices for payment, and which refers to ten months' extraordinary appearances, gives brief details of medication issued (though not always quantity) and cost.

No diagnosis appears on the sheet unless it is in the actual item prescribed. It would also seem that there had been an outbreak of a fever, which was regarded as exceptional for that time.[17]

A bill for various amounts of timber and iron-work for a pump at the Gaol at this time suggests that there was water available within its area. There is also mention of work on the brewhouse door.[18]

Francis Lee was again in attendance in 1731 to cure a sore hand and leg of one prisoner, the broken arm of another and for bleeding a third. How the injuries came about is not mentioned, but there must be the possibility that the treatment of sores was necessitated by the use of fetters.[19] The same Surgeon again treated prisoners in 1732, when his bill was for £1[20] and he was needed to treat both felons and debtors in 1733 in respect of bleeding and surgery when he received the sum of £2.[21]

Complaint was made by the debtor prisoners at the Michaelmas Sessions 1733, although what they complained about was not recorded. Nevertheless two of the Justices of the Peace were desired by the Quarter Sessions Court to visit the Gaol and hear any complaint that was made.[22] It was several months before mention occurs in the Quarter Sessions Books, this time concerning how much of the yearly money that the Gaoler received to feed the felons was actually spent for that purpose. Once again the same two Justices, John Wedgewood and Thomas Abnett, were desired to look into the matter and report back to the Court. No doubt they did, but given the nature of the Court business unless an order had been made as a result of any discussion no record would have been kept. It does indicate, however, that the Justices were not indifferent to the Gaol or its prisoners, but the disciplinary sentiments of the day would have prevailed.[23]

The next record of money paid out on the medical treatment of the prisoners does not occur until 1740, when Phillip Purioll, Surgeon, was allowed £12–0s–8d for sixteen weeks' attendance in the cure of three abscesses on the leg of a prisoner under sentence of transportation, the same man also requiring treatment to a gangrenous buttock.[24] Francis Lee returns again in respect of surgery at the end of the same year, being paid £2–9s–0d for his work.[25]

It is not unreasonable to assume that the expense incurred in the provision of medical treatment for offenders became a subject of discussion between the Justices at their meetings. No doubt the need to keep costs to a minimum may have been argued. That may account for an order of the Court at the Easter Sessions of 1741, stipulating that for the future when any prisoners should be sick in the Gaol and unable to make provision for medical care, then one of the Justices of the Peace, William Robbins, Esq., together with the Clerk of the Peace, Henry Dolphin, were to examine into the truth of the matter and if they judged it necessary were then authorized by the Court to order the Keeper of the Gaol to find and provide a convenient room and bed and all things necessary for that prisoner's subsistence during the continuation of the sickness, reporting to the Court what the Gaoler should reasonably be allowed for such lodging and maintenance, which money was to be raised from the County Stock.[26]

From the next Sessions there was a more regular submission of bills to the Court. Edward Thorley, Apothecary, asked £7–7s–10d for bleeding, attending and administering physic and other medicines to several sick prisoners in the County Gaol.[27] In the following January, Thorley's bill (for a short period he attended regularly and the bills were dealt with more or less on an annual basis) was for £5–6s–3d.[28] A year later the sum was £6–17s–10d.[29] The next bill was for £2–0s–0d[30] and then one for £5–2s–4d.[31] These bills would no doubt have been itemized but have not survived but that at the end of 1745, for £2–4s–0d, has. Edward Thorley dealt with fifteen patients all of whom were prescribed ointment at 1s–0d per pot, although the type of ointment is not given; purging draughts for six of them at 6d each time, while a bottle of drops, at 1s–0d a time, on three occasions was provided for one man who also was prescribed Quick Silver at 2d.[32] Further amounts, again where the itemized bill has not survived, are recorded of £5–8s–0d and £2–12s–6d.[33] Mr Thorley's final bill, delivered at the Epiphany Sessions 1748/9, was for £2–12s–6d but by then Edward Thorley had died.[34]

Job Wetwood now appears as the Apothecary attending the Gaol, his first bill, at Translation 1749, being for £5–8s–5d and again the actual account has not survived.[35] After a slightly longer interval, there was a bill for £7–11s–10d, without details.[36] The next bill was for £12–2s–10d, covering some fifteen months, and gives more details: Ointment and Physic for the Itch (allowing that the prisoners mostly slept on straw, perhaps to be expected); Medicine and cure of Venereal disease; Ointment for Shingles; Treatment for Fever; dressing a contused finger; Abscess on Thigh (which took two months to clear); Ointment for Vermin; various Bleedings; Stomach disorders and Piles.[37]

Job Wetwood's next bill (1754) was for £10–3s–1d and included attention to prisoners in the Stafford House of Correction (hitherto not mentioned in the recording of such expenses).[38]

At the Michaelmas Sessions of 1753 the debtor prisoners complained to the Justices that the windows in the Gaol were out of repair, work to remedy the defects was ordered to be carried out and undertaken by a local glazier.[39] The County also agreed to enlarge the Gaol yard (a courtyard had been made in the Gaol in 1636 but whether this was the same yard, allowing for the enlargements that had taken place, I hesitate to venture) and a lease was taken from the Corporation of Stafford for a garden that adjoined the Gaol, the new piece of land being some 39 yards in length by 14 yards in width. It was also ordered that £136–0s–0d be raised on the County to build a wall to enclose this new area.[40]

The original sum of £20 per year that had been allowed the Gaoler to feed the felons had been varied, at the Easter Sessions of 1742, to what the Gaoler should swear on oath that he had expended, not to exceed one penny per day for each felon. This arose because of the increase in the numbers of persons being committed to the Gaol, the Gaoler having been out of pocket as a result.[41] This sum of one penny per day had also been used to provide the felons with straw to sleep on and keep warm, so at the Michaelmas Sessions of 1754 another increase was allowed, the sum being raised to twopence per day per felon, with only threepence out of this sum being stopped each fortnight for the purpose of buying the straw![42]

Mr Wetwood's next bill, in 1755, was for £13–4s–11d; once again the details are not available.[43] Following this there appears to have been an outbreak of what was known as Gaol Distemper, very possibly a similar complaint to the Fever previously mentioned. To prevent prisoners infecting those in Court when brought to trial, the Hall-keeper was provided with Vinegar, Tobacco, Frankincense, Rum and Pitch with which to wash the hall (presumably using a concoction of these items), while the Gaoler received payment for providing Vinegar and Soap to wash the prisoners before they came up for trial.

For whatever reason another Apothecary, Brooks Crutchley, was now appointed to attend the Gaol and supply medicines and the decision as to whether it was necessary for a prisoner to have a bed when sick was now left to the Apothecary. Only one prisoner was to be in a bed and if the Apothecary thought fit a fire could also be provided. If a bed was provided the Gaoler was to receive one shilling per week for providing it. The final bill submitted by Mr Wetwood and dealt with at the Michaelmas Sessions of 1756, was for £21–9s–8d.[44]

These most recent arrangements for the Gaol appear also to have been extended to the Stafford House of Correction, one woman being ill in that establishment receiving nursing, maintenance and baths, bed and coals for ten weeks at a total cost of £2–12s–8d.[45]

Mr Crutchley's next bill, in 1757, was for £10–4s–4d, no other details,[46] but the next, met in 1758, was for the period July 1757 to July 1758, amounting to £21–3s–8½d and includes date of treatment, details of medicine, name of prisoner and cost of each prescription or attention. The charge for Bleeding was 6d; French Barley, 1d; 2oz Flower of Brimstone, 1½d; Sudorific Powders, 4d each; Rhubarb Bolus, 6d; 1oz Camomile Flower, 2d. Extracting the placenta from one woman was charged at 10s 6d while delivering another was also charged at 10s 6d. He may now have replaced the need for a midwife.[47]

The need for improved ventilation in the Gaol had by now been recognized and to advise on the matter came a person from Worcester, the ventilators installed costing £16–16s–0d. There was also revision of the allowance to the prisoners with provision made for a weekly supply of three hundredweight of coal for the day-dungeon from 1 October to 1 April. The deduction of money for straw ceased and each person that lay in the dungeon was to have a piling of straw a fortnight.[48]

Another bill, from Job Crutchley, for the year ending Translation Sessions, 1759, amounted to £20–8s–3d and again the itemized breakdown has survived but thereafter only the total amounts allowed to be paid by the County are available. There are also entries where the Gaoler has been allowed money for supplying beds for sick prisoners.[49]

Whatever his attendance at the Gaol, Mr Crutchley had complained of loss of business in 1762, and in his stead the Court appointed another Apothecary, a Mr Ward.[50] For the next ten years Mr Ward continued to supply treatment to the prisoners. At the Easter Sessions of 1772, however, the Justices took the step of appointing two persons, John Ward and Thomas Wright, to fulfil the duties for a period of twelve months, year and year about, both of the men being Surgeon and Apothecary.[51] Some months later there was a revision of this order the effect of which was that John Ward continued to perform the duties on his own or to be more precise his was the only name to whom payment was authorized, until 1776, when an Apothecary named Fieldhouse joined him in receiving payment and this continued until 1778 when Richard Hughes, then an Apothecary to the Staffordshire General Infirmary (opened in 1766), was appointed to replace them.[52] Richard Hughes was the first of three generations of Hughes to serve the Gaol, Richard dying from Gaol Fever in early 1793 just before the present Gaol was opened,[53] his son Francis Hughes, a Surgeon, taking over (he in turn followed by Robert Hughes, his son, who continued the family tradition until 1870).[54]

With the appointment of Richard Hughes came a set amount to be paid the Surgeon as a salary, £8–0s–0d each year, with a further sum of £12–0s–0d being paid to the Treasurer of the Staffordshire General Infirmary for such medicine, drugs, etc., as Richard Hughes should think requisite and necessary.[55]

Other events, however, had already begun to influence matters. America, to where so many criminals had been despatched under the mercy of transportation, now plunged into what became the War of Independence. This created the problem of what to do with those prisoners who would in the course of events have been sent there. This problem coincided with the endeavours of John Howard, a Quaker and successful businessman, to improve the situation in the Gaol at Bedford, in which County he had recently been Sheriff, by providing a salary for the Keeper instead of that officer relying on fees. In turn this led Howard to tour the nation's Gaols and Houses of Correction resulting in his publication *The State of the Prisons* (1777) and support from a Member of Parliament, Alexander Popham, and other interested persons, which led to a House of Commons Select Committee and to legislation.[56]

In 1774 there was passed an Act of Parliament which, since sickness and death had become a common danger in the nation's Gaols, had the object of preserving prisoners' lives from 'the malignant fever known as Gaol Distemper': by this Act Justices of the Peace were required to order the walls and ceilings of the several cells and wards, both of debtors and felons, to be scraped and white-washed once in every year; fresh air was to be supplied by means of a hand ventilator; two rooms were to be set aside in each Gaol, one for the men and one for the women, where sick prisoners could be set apart and kept separate from those in health; washing tubs were to be provided that prisoners could be washed before being suffered to leave the Gaol and an experienced Surgeon or Apothecary was to be appointed and was required to report to the Justices at each Quarter Sessions upon the state of the prisoners' health. Clothes were to be provided for the prisoners when the Justices saw occasion; the prisoners were not to be kept underground when it was convenient to do otherwise and there was also to be a latitude to the Justices to make other orders as they thought fit for restoring or preserving the health of the prisoners.[57]

Much of this had already been implemented by the Staffordshire Justices but no doubt the Gaol did not reach the standard that the Act would have made desirable. Howard visited Stafford and considered the Gaol too small for the number of prisoners. There was a court (or airing yard) for debtors and one for felons, although this latter court was too small. The debtors' free-ward was above the male felons' dungeon (where the felons slept) and the ventilator for the dungeon was situated in this debtors' ward, but had been out of repair for a number of years. This dungeon was below ground and had no windows and was described as being very close. The women had a separate dungeon. There was a small day-room for both men and women felons. The dungeons had a plentiful supply of clean straw of which Mr Howard approved. Outside the walls of the Gaol there was a small stream; this he regretted was not within the walls, the comment perhaps inferring that the water supply was insufficient. The Gaoler was licensed for beer and wine (this was one of the means whereby the Gaoler gained his subsistence). There was a small chapel at the top of the house.[58]

Howard's observations appear to have eventually had some effect for at a later date the ventilator was provided with a new fan and from the Midsummer period of 1787 the diet of the prisoners was amended to allow milk and potatoes, although the cost of these items was to be found by reducing the amount of bread and cheese previously allowed, so that the expense on the County was not increased. This applied to the prisoners in both the Gaol and the House of Correction.[59]

Following upon the thinking of the day and to remedy the situation that had arisen in law from the abandonment of transportation to the Americas, another Act of Parliament was passed in 1779, providing for the erection of Penitentiary Houses in the London area, where prisoners could be employed at hard labour and lodged in separate rooms. There was temporary accommodation of prisoners who were considered suitable for transportation, aboard ships or vessels, to be kept to work at hard labour dredging rivers or ports and making provision for the transportation of prisoners to other places than the Americas.[60] There was also revision of the laws pertaining to Houses of Correction and another Act, of 1782, rendered it necessary for a new establishment to be provided. Such matters, however, took time. It was necessary for the Stafford County Justices to procure an Act of Parliament to erect a new Gaol and this they did, work commencing in 1787, under the supervision of Commissioners appointed from the Justices, this Gaol being taken into use in May 1793.[61]

The new Gaol comprised a Gaol, House of Correction and Penitentiary for both male and female prisoners. It was a substantial construction of two long buildings parallel to each other, having a ground floor and two upper storeys, the two buildings being linked in two places on each level so as to provide access throughout, with the spaces between the buildings providing an inner and two outer courtyards, with various yards at the front and rear, all of which were secured by palings. The different categories of prisoners were kept separate. Set in the centre of the building facing the Gate-lodge which gave entrance to the Gaol, was the house for the Governor who was required to live in the Gaol (and who now served as both Keeper of the Gaol and Master of the House of Correction). These buildings and yards were surrounded by a high boundary wall in the centre of which, facing the road, was the Gate-lodge.[62]

The Surgeon, Francis Hughes, was allowed £15–0s–0d per year for his services, with another £15–0s–0d being paid to the General Infirmary for the supply of drugs and medicines, etc. His duties were to visit any prisoners who were kept in the sick ward once every day and to see all other prisoners once a week. He was to attend the prison immediately if the Governor advised of any new sickness, or in the case of a new prisoner who in the opinion of the Governor required examination before being allowed into the prison proper (the Gate-lodge which had reception rooms and various small facilities was technically not part of the prison at that stage, but prisoners considered contagious could be kept there apart from others until seen by the Surgeon). The Surgeon was to keep a Journal (this does not appear to have been done, certainly not in the early years) and report to the Justices at each Quarter Sessions of the Peace as to the state of the prisoners under his care. If in the opinion of the Surgeon any wine or spirituous liquor was essential for the health of any prisoner then such medication could not be allowed unless the prisoner was removed to the sick ward beforehand. The Surgeon was also allowed to authorize the issue of extra bedding, clothing or food.[63]

Mention of spirituous liquors deserves comment. These had been prohibited in the Gaols of the country since circa 1751, but beer had not (the supply of water available may have been unreliable and perhaps improved by the process of brewing) while some of the debtor prisoners would have desired wine from time to time. The supply of beer was still considered, in some areas, to be an essential part of the Gaoler's means of living. This last matter was remedied in 1784, when legislation was passed authorizing the Justices of the Peace to allow the Gaoler a salary in lieu of the profits derived from the sale of liquor.[64] At Stafford the Justices did so in 1785, the then Governor receiving a salary of £100 per year.[65] It is worth mentioning that the Keepers of the Houses of Correction in the County had been prohibited from selling strong liquors or keeping an ale-house in their House in 1745.[66]

The opening of the new County Gaol virtually brings to an end the period under review, but the turn of the century brought the first legislation to attempt to deal properly with the problem of insanity. Influencing this was the illness suffered by George the Third and which led to the Regency period. There was also the attempt that had been made on the life of the King by a man named Hadfield bringing with it a trial for treason. Before then, where those so afflicted fell foul of the law it appears to have been a matter for the judgement of those in charge of the Courts. As early as 1749/50 a man brought before the Staffordshire Quarter Sessions on charges relating to the Vagrancy laws was deemed to be a lunatic and ordered to be kept in the House of Correction at the charge of the County, as he seemed incapable of working for his maintenance, and remained there until he died in 1755. The regular sums paid for his maintenance, including such clothing as was necessary, would have ensured that he was not altogether forgotten, but there is nothing to indicate how he was treated by those in whose charge he remained.[67] An Act of Parliament passed in 1740, dealing with Rogues and Vagabonds, refers to 'persons of little or no estates, who by their lunacy or otherwise, are furiously mad, or so far disordered in their senses, that they may be dangerous to be permitted to go abroad' and the Justices were required to cause such person(s) to be apprehended and kept safely locked up in some secure place within the County or place and if found necessary 'to be there chained'.[68] The places most readily available to the County Justices were the Gaol and Houses of Correction, although it is possible that Parish officials could find other accommodation.

Finally, the new Gaol, in relation to that which it replaced, must then have seemed a huge building affording far superior conditions than anything that Stafford had previously enjoyed. The sleeping cells were of two sizes, 9' x 8' 6' or 7' x 6', all being 8' 6' high and were arranged in arcade fashion either side of a central passageway. They had two doors, an iron grated door for security and a wooden door that could be closed over. The windows of the cells had wooden shutters that could be closed when the weather was inclement (the debtors had glass windows but this was not extended to the other categories until later). The prisoners were not to remain in their cells during the day-time, unless specially permitted by the Governor; there were various 'day-rooms' set aside. Those convicted were required to work, the hours of labour being adjusted to the time of year, although the supply of work was not always regular. There was also variation between the different categories of prisoners. Sanctions were authorized against those prisoners that offended against the rules.[69]

Prisoners under sentence of death were kept apart from other prisoners, prisoners sentenced to death for wilful murder were then by law executed the day but one after sentence was passed, unless that day was a Sunday or Holy day when sentence would have been carried out the day after that. For them there was no provision for exercise; diet was bread and water; they were not allowed visitors, unless by the written permission of the Trial-Judge, Sheriff or Under-Sheriff. Sentence of death for other offences did admit of minor privileges.[70]

If a debtor prisoner was taken ill he could have his wife attend him in the sick-ward, subject to the Governor's permission.[71] There was no provision for female staff to supervise the female prisoners. Sanitary arrangements were not recorded but it is known that at a slightly later date 'privvy' areas existed in the yards and it is not unreasonable to assume that this was the situation when the Gaol opened. The Infirmary area did not have a water closet anywhere near it, a matter that was not taken up by the Justices until some twenty years later.[72] Substantial though the new Prison may have been, it was very soon the subject of constant amendment, additional buildings and alterations.

During the course of the eighteenth century the Gaol at Stafford had undergone structural improvement, although details are vague. Medical treatment of prisoners had begun, initially in a selective manner (i.e. those for transportation) then extending to all of the prisoners in the Gaol and House of Correction; from the visit of the Apothecary or Surgeon as occasion demanded to the appointment of a regular Surgeon, salaried with an additional supply of medicines. The original Gaol seems to have been without rooms that could be permanently set aside for sick prisoners, but this was remedied with the new Gaol. The confinement of many prisoners together in a large chamber had given way to improved conditions, which afforded some separation of the different classes of prisoners. The provision of food had improved. The financial security of the Gaoler, guaranteed by a salary, removed his need to supply liquor to the prisoners as a means of support, while the County had taken over the payment of his assistants. The role of the Chaplain, while remaining a part-time post, was extended with the new Gaol, being provided with a chapel and required to see each prisoner privately and observe the state of the cells. While in the old Gaol there was no provision of work for the prisoners, now a Taskmaster was to be appointed and all categories of convicted prisoners required to work and others encouraged to do so. A step forward had been made in the treatment of prisoners.

Notes

1. SRO MFQ3 Easter 1720. This reference specifies a midwife attending in the House of Correction. Expenses to the Gaoler at various times back to the turn of the century leave little room for doubt that the amount included services other than just food and warmth.
2. After Ann was executed the child was removed to the Parish of Albington, Shropshire, the last place of settlement of the murdered father, Thomas Davenhill. The Gaoler's expenses totalled £3–6s–6d. SRO MFQ2 Easter 1703.
3. SRO QSR/402 Michaelmas 1686.
4. SRO MFQ2 Easter 1706.
5. SRO MFQ2 Michaelmas 1699 and QSMe/1 f64.
6. SRO MFQ4 Epiphany 1767. This allowance was for those prisoners committed for a period of twelve months. There had earlier been provision for those considered incapable of supporting themselves.
7. 23 Henry VIII, cap 2: 'An Act concerning where and under what manner the Gaols within this Realm shall be edified and made'.
8. The Victoria History of the County of Stafford, vol. VI (Oxford University Press, 1979), 271, para 9. When the new Gaol was opened at Stafford in 1793 a charity box to receive contributions from the public was fixed at the gate. Money collected was ordered to be used according to the directions of a committee formed by the Sheriff, Visiting Justices, Chaplain and Surgeon. A. J. Standley, 'Stafford Gaol 1793–1916', 6, (unpublished, William Salt Library, Stafford).
9. Victoria History of Staffordshire, vol. VI (Oxford University Press, 1979), 203, 204; and SRO D/1323/E/1/f20 and f36. The Town appears to have still had its own Gaol circa 1695 (WSL (uncat) Norbury 35).
10. SRO MFQ1 Trinity 1620 and Epiphany 1621/22. Also SRO MFQ2 Translation 1687 and Michaelmas 1696.
11. SRO QSMe/1 f133 and 138; SRO MFQ3 Michaelmas 1714 and Easter 1715.
12. SRO QSMe/1 f209 and MFQ3 Michaelmas 1727.
13. SRO MFQ3 Epiphany 1727/8. 4 George 1, cap 11: 'An Act for the further preventing Robbery, Burglary, and other Felonies, and for the more effectual Transportation of Felons, and unlawful exporters of Wool; and for Declaring the law upon some points relating to Piracy'.
14. SRO MFQ3 Translation 1729.
15. SRO MFQ3 Epiphany 1729/30.
16. SRO QSBm 12.
17. See above. This outbreak of fever affected many prisoners and appears to have been the earliest at Stafford, during this period, to receive mention, two other serious outbreaks occurring in 1757 and 1793 (see below, notes 44 and 54). While the exact conditions prevailing in

the Gaol are not clear, there seems little cause to doubt that in most Gaols fever was endemic, perhaps many prisoners developing some resistance, but that a more virulent form might cause an outbreak from time to time. See *Gentleman's Magazine*, May 1750, 235; Basil Williams, *The Whig Supremacy* (Oxford: Oxford University Press, 1962), 135–6; C. P. Hill, *British Economic and Social History, 1700–1939* (London: Edward Arnold Ltd, 1964).

18. SRO MFQ3 Michaelmas 1730 and QSBe 32.
19. SRO MFQ3 Epiphany 1731/32.
20. SRO MFQ3 Translation 1732.
21. SRO MFQ3 Easter 1733.
22. SRO MFQ3 Michaelmas 1733. The selection of these two Justices for the task was by reason that they lived near to the Gaol. It is easy in this day and age to lose sight of the fact that many of the Justices lived in more distant parts of the County, sometimes several hours' travel away.
23. SRO MFQ3 Translation 1734.
24. SRO MFQ4 Easter 1740.
25. SRO MFQ4 Epiphany 1740/1.
26. SRO MFQ4 Easter 1741.
27. SRO MFQ4 Translation 1741.
28. SRO MFQ4 Epiphany 1741/2.
29. SRO MFQ4 Epiphany 1742/3.
30. SRO MFQ4 Michaelmas 1743.
31. SRO MFQ4 Epiphany 1744/5.
32. SRO MFQ4 Michaelmas 1745 and QSBe 15.
33. SRO MFQ4 Michaelmas 1746 and Easter 1748. There is additionally another bill for £1–7s–6d that I have inadvertently omitted in the script. Translation 1747.
34. SRO MFQ4 Epiphany 1748/9.
35. SRO MFQ4 Translation 1749.
36. SRO MFQ4 Epiphany 1751/2.
37. SRO MFQ4 Translation 1752 and QSBe 19/13.
38. SRO MFQ4 Epiphany 1754. It may be relevant that at this time there was a prisoner in the House of Correction at Stafford confined as a lunatic and maintained at the expense of the County.
39. SRO MFQ4 Michaelmas 1753 and Translation 1754.
40. SRO MFQ4 Michaelmas 1753; Translation and Michaelmas 1754.
41. SRO MFQ4 Easter 1742.
42. SRO MFQ4 Michaelmas 1754.
43. SRO MFQ4 Translation 1755.
44. SRO MFQ4 Easter 1756.
45. SRO MFQ4 Epiphany 1757.
46. SRO MFQ4 Translation 1757.
47. SRO MFQ4 Translation 1758 and QSBe 22/13.
48. SRO MFQ4 Easter and Michaelmas 1758. The man from Worcester

was Richard Blackwell.

49. SRO MFQ4 Translation 1759. Before the coal allowance was granted the Gaoler also received payment for coal that he had supplied the prisoners when sick.
50. SRO MFQ4 Easter 1762.
51. SRO MFQ5 Easter 1772.
52. SRO MFQ5 Translation 1776.
53. Burial Register, St Mary's, Stafford, March 1793.
54. A. J. Standley, 'Stafford Gaol, 1793–1916', 2, 119, 120, 180 (WSL, unpublished).
55. SRO MFQ5 Epiphany 1778.
56. 14 Geo III, cap 20: 'An Act for the Relief of Prisoners charged with felony, or other Crimes, who shall be acquitted or discharged by Proclamation, respecting the Payment of Fees to Gaolers, and giving a recompense for such Fees out of the County Rates'; see also Roy Porter's essay in this volume.
57. 14 Geo III, cap 59: 'An Act for Preserving the Health of Prisoners in Gaol and Preventing the Gaol Distemper'.
58. J. Howard, *An Account of the present state of the Prisons in the Oxford Circuit* (London, 1789), 29–32.
59. Staffordshire Treasurer's Account Book 1787–1830, William Salt Library.
60. 19 Geo III, cap 74: 'An Act to explain and amend the laws relating to the Transportation, Imprisonment, and other punishment of certain offenders'.
61. 27 Geo III, cap 60: 'An Act for building a new Gaol, and providing a proper Prison for Debtors, and House of Correction, for the several Boroughs, Towns Corporate, Liberties, Franchises, and all other Places, within the County of Stafford; and for regulating the same respectively'. The prison was built to the design of William Blackburn. *The Victoria History of the County of Stafford*, vol. VI (Oxford University Press, 1979), 232, and A. J. Standley, 'Stafford Gaol 1793–1916', 6/7 (WSL, unpublished).
62. A. J. Standley, 'Stafford Gaol 1793–1916', 1 (WSL, unpublished).
63. See above, page 3.
64. 24 Geo III, cap 54: 'An Act to amend and explain the Act of 11/12 William III cap 19 (An Act to enable Justices of the Peace to build and repair Gaols in their respective Counties)'.
65. SRO MFQ6 Michaelmas 1785.
66. SRO MFQ4 Michaelmas 1745.
67. William Markway was confined in the House of Correction at Stafford from 7 November 1749 until his death in 1755 during which time there was regular money paid the Keeper for Markway's maintenance. He was buried at St Mary's, Stafford on 17 June, 1755.
68. 13 George 11: 'An Act to amend the laws relating to Rogues and Vagabonds'.

69. SRO MFQ6 Epiphany 1793: 'Rules, Orders and Regulations for the government of the Gaol'.
70. See above and 25 Geo 11, cap 37: 'An Act for the better preventing the horrid crime of murder'.
71. SRO MFQ6 Epiphany 1793: 'Rules, Orders and Regulations for the government of the Gaol'.
72. A. J. Standley, 'Stafford Gaol 1793–1916', 52 (WSL, unpublished).

SRO = Stafford Records Office.
WSL = William Salt Library, (Reference), Stafford.
MFQ = Microfilm

3

The Health of Prisoners and the Two Faces of Benthamism

Martin J. Wiener

What is the place of Benthamism in the history of British prisons? This is a more difficult question than it would have been a generation ago; in recent years the association once freely made of Bentham and his followers with every manifestation of state rationalization and expansion in the nineteenth century has been severely qualified by scholars.[1] There were many sources of new social and political thinking in that era of great mental ferment besides Jeremy Bentham. As M. J. Cullen remarked some years ago, 'it is time that historians stopped calling any middle-class intellectual with a coherent social ideology a Benthamite'.[2] By now that injunction has been taken to heart by historians, and our picture of the mental environment surrounding the rise of modern British social administration has expanded and diversified considerably. In particular, we have come to see the archetypically Benthamite impatience with waste and disorder, and accompanying confidence in what could be achieved through the rationalization of institutional life – so important for the development of modern prisons – as emerging from the late eighteenth century onward in the activities and arguments of a considerable number of persons, starting for prisons perhaps with John Howard; a procession in which Bentham was, however important, only one figure.

Nonetheless, Bentham and Utilitarianism retain, justifiably, a pre-eminent place in the history of social administration in modern Britain, and specifically in that of penal policy. Bentham's philosophy, as Elie Halevy pointed out many years ago, was distinctive in being a philosophy written for men engaged in governing.[3] And in fact, his systematic, comprehensive and voluminous writings, taken up by remarkably intelligent and energetic followers, did indeed shape a climate of thinking about the purposes of government, the character of social problems and forms of public policy that influenced many persons in or around social administration who may never have read a word of Bentham. These writings, moreover, as we shall see, created a vocabulary in which continuing problems of penal administration were to be discussed from his time down to ours.

In a strict sense, British prisons were never Benthamite. Not only because they were never put under private contractors, as Bentham proposed in his Panopticon plan, and not only because no prison was ever built on strict Panopticon physical lines, where all inmates would be under surveillance at all times. More generally, if not surprisingly, the purely 'rational' and 'scientific' institutions Bentham envisioned were never realized. Instead, like judicial proceedings, prisons were always shaped more by politics than by science, more by 'sentiment' (both tender and harsh) than by impassive rationality.

Yet, in a less purist sense, British prisons were deeply Benthamite, for the official definitions of their tasks, administration and procedures borrowed heavily from Bentham. The new sort of middle-class professional involved in defining, inspecting and running prisons – 'statist' politicians, social scientists, civil servants and medical men – all found Utilitarian discourse a natural fit, an attractive counterbalance to the inevitable pressures of politics and sentiment.

The very term, Benthamism, is rather misleading, for it presumes *a* Benthamism, one harmonious set of ideals. In fact, Bentham's Utilitarianism contained many divergent inclinations and inner tensions and contestations, themselves rooted in the Enlightenment, from which Benthamism of course derived. For example, 'penal Benthamism', with which we are particularly concerned today, was different in many significant respects from Benthamism as a general socio-political philosophy. The scope of Benthamite government, as a general rule, was to be limited by the principle that each man was normally the best judge of what would conduce to his own happiness. Government's role was to provide the framework of security and predictability within which individuals could pursue their own happiness, not to prescribe the forms that happiness was to take. Moreover, Bentham's suspicion of personal interest led him to equip his governmental model with far-reaching controls upon the unbridled exercise of administrative power, notably wide publicity and frequent democratic elections.[4] Penal Benthamism, on the other hand, was decidedly more interventionist and authoritarian. Obviously, its subjects – criminal offenders – were there for purposes other than pursuing their happiness or interest (indeed, it was for the interest of the rest of society that they were incarcerated). Less obviously but just as importantly, prisoners were exceptions to the general Benthamite rule just cited that each man was the best judge of his own interests. Criminal offenders were different from normal people. Bentham described 'delinquents' as 'a peculiar race of beings, who require unremitted inspection. Their weakness consists in yielding to the seductions of the passing moment. Their minds are weak and disordered.'[5] It was largely *because* of their defectiveness in personal cost-benefit analysis that they had fallen afoul of the law, so until their characters were changed (which he had high hopes of doing), they would require firm and extensive management from outside. Such a requirement readily merged with the growing confidence in what could be achieved through the rationalization of institutional life to produce the kind of almost totalitarian visions so acutely criticized by both conservatives and radicals in our own day. From very different standpoints, Gertrude Himmelfarb and Michel Foucault have (not entirely justly) made Bentham's Panopticon prison plan synonymous with Orwellian surveillance and manipulation.[6] Even if Himmelfarb and Foucault must be taken with several grains of salt – and they must – it is undoubtedly true that 'Benthamite ideals' in relation to prisons and prisoners operated at some remove from, even in some tension with, Benthamism or Utilitarianism as a general philosophy. Thus, the subject of this essay has to be considered as a *special* case of Benthamism or Utilitarianism.

Nor was penal Benthamism itself unitary and conflict-free. Indeed, an inescapable tension, one centrally relevant to the question of the health of prisoners, ran through it: that between punishment and care. It is true, and important to note, that the conflict between these two tasks was for the nineteenth century less than it might seem to us. In a society of comparatively low living standards, where hardship and deprivation were normal experiences, quite harsh prison conditions were not difficult to justify, and not necessarily perceived as cruel. Indeed, reformation, an important and practicable goal for Benthamites, with their picture of human behaviour as comparatively malleable, was itself seen, in a way most people today would find almost perverse, as an inherently painful process. Benthamites frequently described the hedonistic calculus in Evangelical-like terms of struggle; as the economist Nassau Senior observed in 1836, 'to abstain from the enjoyment which is in our power, or to seek distant rather than immediate results, are among the most painful [and necessary] exertions of the human will'.[7]

Yet, even taking into account these 'Victorian' elements of Benthamism, there remained in it an irreducible degree of tension between two legitimate and necessary tasks of penal institutions. On one hand, the fundamental purpose of punishment was to prevent future offences by example, that is, deterrence – this was, Bentham remarked, 'beyond comparison the most important' of the ends of penal policy.[8] Deterrence of course involved the infliction of pain. Yet in a hedonistic and individualistic philosophy like Utilitarianism, any infliction of pain upon individuals without their consent requires strong justification ('all punishment is mischief; all punishment in itself is evil'),[9] in this case by its prevention of the greater pains of future offences. Thus, deterrent punishment must be limited to the minimum amount necessary to achieve its effect on future behaviour, of the offender himself and, more important, of potential offenders; any 'unnecessary' suffering is an illegitimate use of power. The essence of Bentham's approach was a never-ending effort to keep these two claims upon the policymaker in balance, and not let either 'punitive' or 'humanitarian' considerations rule. Bentham himself realized that it was not an enterprise likely to satisfy many observers: 'Some [he admonished] forget that a convict in prison is a sensitive being; others, that he is put there for punishment.'[10] Ironically, this philosophy so natural to bureaucrats was at the same time particularly hard on the agents of authority: if they inflicted either too little or too much punishment they had failed in their responsibility. Benthamism prescribed the diminution of crime as a basic responsibility of government, but it also *pro*scribed the causing of, or – even more important for the health of prisoners – the failing to prevent, unnecessary and avoidable harm to offenders.

Specifically, Bentham set out three principles by which the treatment of incarcerated criminal offenders was to be guided. First, the 'rule of lenity' prescribed that the 'ordinary condition' of convicted prisoners should not involve gratuitous physical suffering or danger to health or life. This rule stood against retributive passions, against any infliction of pain that did not yield clear and proportionate results in general well-being, and even against neglect (the pains of omission, so typical of eighteenth-century imprisonment). It also had direct bearing on questions of health, for it suggested that the prison authorities had a duty to allow no preventable injury or illness. As medical and administrative capabilities developed, the sphere of what was seen as preventable expanded, and this rule would similarly expand the obligations of prison authorities.

However, against this tendency stood Bentham's second rule, the 'rule of severity', that prisoners' condition 'ought not to be made more eligible than that of the poorest class of subjects in a state of innocence and liberty'. This rule of 'less eligibility' stemmed from the fact that the prisoners were after all there chiefly as a deterrent to further crime. In regard to health, it qualified the first rule, tending to limit the duty of care to that level of health enjoyed by the general population. For if prisoners were to receive the best health care the state could provide, it would be difficult to prevent their condition from becoming more eligible than that of poor free labourers in a society where such care was a very scarce good.

The second rule was reinforced by a third, the 'rule of economy', that 'saving the regard due to life, health, bodily ease, proper instruction, and future provision, economy ought, in every point of management, to be the prevalent consideration'.[11] Any expenditure beyond that necessary to follow the first two rules represented a waste of social resources that could have been otherwise employed to increase the sum total of happiness.

These rules exhibited the two sides, both legitimate, of penal Benthamism, the first focusing on the 'humanitarian' and the latter two on the 'punitive'. These two faces were neither completely separable nor reconcilable. In the continual and inescapable tension between them lay the ongoing dilemma of prison health care. Between the state's responsibility to keep the situation of prisoners 'less eligible' than the poorest free citizens and the state's equal responsibility to preserve prisoners' lives and health, a permanent process of struggle and negotiation ensued, both between prisoners and their keepers, and among the keepers themselves. The first type of struggle – between prisoners and prison authorities – has recently been highlighted by scholars, inspired practically by prisoners' rights movements and theoretically by Foucault.[12] This essay will focus on the second type of struggle – among the keepers – and on the degree to which it was carried on *within* as well as between keepers. For it should be clear that the conflict was not simply between 'good' and 'bad' authorities, or even 'good' and 'bad' principles, but also (and perhaps more fundamentally) between two equally basic aspects of one philosophy.

Each aspect did have its own particular professional appeal. Medical men, especially academics and those involved in the public health movement, whose professional reason for being was the diminution of ill health and suffering, responded most readily to the rule of lenity. Criminal justice administrators, from judges to Home Office civil servants to prison governors, tended to place the rules of severity and economy in lead position. Medical men who also played administrative roles – prison medical officers – were caught between these stances. Prison medical officers in the nineteenth century (and to a degree, still today) had a highly complex and difficult job, carrying out an essentially Benthamite task of balancing the demands of these three rules of lenity, severity and economy. For they could never forget that they were supplying health care services, free of charge (in an age when everyone else had to pay for their medical care), to a population under sentence of punishment for criminal offences against the public that was paying for their care. From another angle, they were combining, and mediating between, two faces of practical Benthamism – what we might call a 'positive' or 'welfare' face, that of the new public health movement, seeking to provide through government collective provision for needs that were not being met individually, and a 'negative' or 'punitive' face, that of the new system of workhouses and prisons, seeking to provide also through government needed sanctions that were not being provided against individuals for their anti-social behaviour in society at large.

This tension existed from the early days of both public health and 'institutional discipline'. It was evident in the clash over prison conditions of two pioneers of public health – Edwin Chadwick, author of the landmark *Report on the Sanitary Condition of the Labouring Population* (1842), and William Farr, who had been hired in 1837, with Chadwick's recommendation, by the newly-created General Registry Office, becoming in 1839 its chief statistician. Chadwick and Farr had many views in common; in particular, both crusaded for a national Board of Health.[13] As secretary of the Poor Law Commission, seeking to establish national standards for workhouse dietaries, Chadwick had examined the dietaries of sixty gaols. He divided the gaols into three classes of twenty each, 'lowest', 'intermediate' and 'full'. By comparing illness and death in each class, he was able to argue not only that lenity and economy were not necessarily opposed, but that in fact as a class the gaols with the lowest dietary had also the lowest mortality.[14] In this imaginative statistical operation Chadwick made a basic error: to generate morbidity and mortality rates, he had used the more easily available figures of committals rather than the more relevant datum of the actual average gaol population. This was pointed out to him privately soon after,[15] but Chadwick, as was his wont when challenged, stuck by his dubious procedure,[16] and became ever more identified over the next few years with an 'economical' position on workhouse and gaol provision, usually finding local conditions long on diet and short on labour.[17] Several years later a far more damaging, because public, criticism of his statistical 'experiment' appeared in the reformist medical journal, *The Lancet*, authored anonymously by Farr.[18] Farr made a number of complaints about Chadwick's collection of information, finding for example a highly incomplete notation of medical complaints in low-dietary gaols. As an emerging authority on statistics, however, Farr focused his critique on Chadwick's interpretive procedures, patronizingly observing that 'the data [had] been ingeniously collected, but inaccurately interpreted'. Using committals rather than average gaol population was an error with dramatic consequences, for 'prisoners on the lowest dietaries ... were detained only thirty-four days; while in the gaols with what he has called "full dietaries", they remain eighty-two days on an average'.[19] Once corrected for actual days spent, the higher death and disease rates of full dietary gaols more than disappeared. Moreover, Farr went on to make a general criticism of prison conditions, noting that in simply comparing gaol mortality, Chadwick had ignored the high rate of overall gaol mortality – 'nearly double the mortality of the country population at the same age'.[20]

Chadwick and Farr were to clash again over public health statistical methods,[21] but the fundamental issue between them was less a matter of scientific technique[22] and more one of how they defined their task. While the two men were both strong 'environmentalists' in regard to public health, they sharply differed on questions of prisoners' health. For Farr, a doctor, prisons were merely one more social environment, indeed as a manmade environment, one peculiarly open to human control; thus for him *any* excess in prison morbidity or mortality over that of a comparable non-prison population constituted an indictment of their administration.[23]

This was not so for Chadwick, trained not in medicine but in law and engaged in constructing new forms of social administration. Chadwick, unlike Farr, was concerned equally with two forms of 'social health': physical and moral. Despite the critical role he was coming to see environment playing in explaining disparities in mortality between differing locales in the country at large, Chadwick made a sharp distinction between the 'penal' and the non-penal population; in contrast to the general public environment, the prison (like the workhouse) had to serve several purposes simultaneously – Bentham's lenity, severity and economy.[24] From his standpoint, to examine the health of prisoners in isolation from other penal questions was sentimental and one-sided, un-Benthamite, and sure to yield bad penal policy. Indeed, if Farr saw only the duty to protect the prisoner's health, in Chadwick's field of vision this duty had to jostle for space with sterner obligations. By the time of their quarrel Chadwick already had come to disapprove of the use of lengthy imprisonment as a penal measure precisely because misguided reformers were making prison conditions too comfortable, and thus neither economical nor deterrent. Instead, he recommended short terms of imprisonment, with separate confinement wherever practicable, followed by extensive periods of police surveillance.[25] Moreover, Chadwick liked to point out that 'prisoners when brought in are not a healthy class', and that they are often 'discharged in greater health and strength than when they came in'.[26] Farr, on the other hand, tended to see imprisonment as in itself physically injurious, 'lowering the spirits', requiring positive countermeasures; he also opposed lengthy imprisonment, but for the opposite reason from Chadwick – its almost inevitable damage to health.[27]

Although Chadwick had the Benthamite credentials, in a larger sense, Farr also represented a wider, more diffuse Benthamism – a vision of indefinite improvement in social well-being through the application of scientific advances and more generally through rational administration of public affairs by professional experts. Farr exemplified the outlook of many in the rising medical profession, particularly those involved in public health activities. These two faces of Benthamism were joined in the new role of prison medical officer, established by law in 1774 but only becoming institutionalized with the early Victorian reconstruction, rationalization and expansion of prisons. The reports of these officers continually negotiate the tensions between the two imperatives of Benthamism.

Perhaps the foremost prison medical officer of the mid-Victorian period was William Guy,[28] no mere functionary but an eminent member of the medical profession. He became Medical Superintendant of Millbank Prison, *de facto* senior prison medical officer,[29] in 1859 after serving for some years as Dean of the medical faculty at King's College, London, and before that as Professor of Forensic Medicine there. He was also a public health activist, taking part in founding the Health of Towns Association and, as the *Dictionary of National Biography* noted, 'incessantly occupied in calling public attention to questions of sanitary reform by investigations (statistical and medical), lectures, and writings'.[30] In 1869, after resigning from the prison system, he was appointed Professor of Hygiene at King's College. His public health activism was supported by expertise as a statistician: he was editor of the *Journal of the Statistical Society* from 1852 to 1856 and President of the Statistical Society in 1873–5.

Guy's public role was as both a humanitarian and a scientist.[31] He saw himself following in the footsteps of John Howard, about whom he wrote a book and delivered several papers. One of his first actions as

President of the Statistical Society was to get a Howard medal established, to be regularly awarded, to permanently enshrine Howard's position, not just as a prison reformer, but as a pioneer of social statistics. Guy's Howard was a founder of modern *scientific* humanitarianism, or, as he put it, 'preventive philanthropy'.[32] Indeed, in Guy's description Howard sounded very much like Chadwick's Bentham – 'founder of a new method of procedure in matters social' and no less than 'the inaugurator of a new epoch in the history of England and the world'.[33] Howard 'set the first example of that method of procedure in bringing about the reform of abuses [publicity, investigation, legislation, inspection] which the people and Government of England now resort to on every suitable occasion'.[34] In particular, the Government, for, as Guy concluded one address, Howard 'taught us of how much wrong and suffering the State, by omission or commission, can become the direct cause'.[35]

Guy has recently been sharply criticized as a leading betrayer of his calling by placing the health needs of his prison patients below pennypinching punitiveness. His evidence to the 1863 Carnarvon Committee on Prisons, and the recommendations of the 1864 Committee on Prison Dietaries chaired by him – which included reductions in the amount and variety of food allowed most prisoners – have been cited by modern historians for their callousness.[36] This criticism, while not false, must be placed in historiographical context. From heroes of earlier Whiggish histories of penal progress, prison medical officers have become villains in the accounts of penal failure by critical revisionists. However, while such revisionism has exposed just how blinkered the 'humanitarian' interpretation of penal history has been, revisionists have often donned blinkers of their own, in assuming that the only proper role for the prison medical officer was oppositional, to put forth the claims of 'care' against 'punishment'. Ironically, despite rhetorical ties to post-structuralism, most revisionists seem to have missed the post-structural critique of simplistic binary oppositions. Instead of either celebrating the humanity or indicting the inhumanity of prison medicine, this paper suggests a more nuanced and complex interpretation that takes account of the *multiplicity* of legitimate purposes guiding most prison medical officers in general, and Guy in particular, a multiplicity best grasped in the context of the Utilitarian legacy.

We can best understand Guy and prison medical officers in general in the nineteenth century by seeing them as Utilitarians, bearing particular responsibility for one social aim – health – but aware that it had ultimately to be balanced against other, equally legitimate, social aims. Guy, for example, was a genuine enthusiast for the continual improvement of public health through medical progress and state activism, while at the same time, as regards the penal system, striving to balance the Benthamite principles of lenity, severity and economy. He was a strong advocate of increased medical authority in prisons, and argued for basing prison health policies on the best scientific knowledge available rather than on tradition, vested interests or popular prejudices. He helped abolish scurvy in prisons by seeing that all prisoners were supplied with potatoes; he undertook personal investigations which cast doubt on prevailing beliefs that local prison diet was markedly higher than that of free labourers; he warned the Carnarvon Committee on Prisons against hasty tampering with the dietary;[37] and he defended the authority of the medical officer to alter diet and even interfere with punishments, in individual cases, on grounds of health. Yet he also proposed the removal of meat from dietaries; agreed that, in contrast to local prisons, the dietaries of *convict* prisons were excessive; invidiously contrasted the unhealthy living conditions soldiers were expected to endure (conditions he had a few years earlier investigated) with the more generous situation of convicts; and insisted that while the medical officer should never inflict punishment he 'should so perform his functions as to promote the discipline of the prison',[38] using restraint and even, if necessary, diet as disciplinary tools, and strictly limiting his exercise of the power of exempting individual prisoners from the usual disciplinary regime.[39]

The key to these apparent contradictions is the Benthamite balancing calculus between punishment and care. A prisoner (especially a convict) was for Guy a very special kind of patient, one who had seriously harmed his fellow-citizens; his punishment was socially and morally as necessary as his care. In arguing, as a medical man, in defence of the insanity plea, he disclaimed the bias towards leniency that tended to be associated with this position:

> I have always felt more sympathy with the victims, than with the perpetrators, of crime; I do not shrink from the thought of the pain inflicted by corporal punishment when it falls on cruel and brutal offenders against the law, or on those who add serious breaches of prison discipline to the crimes which led to their incarceration; nor have I found any reason to prefer any other punishment for murder to death upon the scaffold.[40]

In order to scientifically settle the arguments about the health of prisoners, he conducted a census of the entire convict population in

1861 and found that 'the rate of mortality of male convicts, when calculated in the manner least open to exception, and compared with the best standards we possess, was highly favourable, and that of female convicts far from unsatisfactory'. The convict death rate (*contra* Farr) was thus in Guy's estimation not higher than for comparable populations outside. Indeed, 'when we consider that the greater part of the convict population belongs to that class of society which occupies by choice, and almost of necessity, the worst localities and the worst residences of our towns, large and small, and of our most populous villages, we should probably be selecting a more just standard of comparison, if, instead of England and London, we took as our standard the worst districts of the metropolis'.

As far as prisons were concerned, he concluded, 'the work which John Howard set himself to do seems to have been fully accomplished'. These institutions were as healthy as – given their special functions and their special population – one could reasonably expect them to be:

> The prisoner not only undergoes no punishment beyond that which the law awards him, or which his own perverse conduct in prison may bring upon him; not only is he not exposed to the gaol fever, the small-pox, and other fatal maladies, which decimated our prisons less than a century ago, but his health is carefully protected against every cause of injury not inseparable from the state of imprisonment and his own wilful misconduct when in prison.[41]

This was not to say, Guy acknowledged, that prisons were an ideal health environment, but that was in the nature of imprisonment, which obviously had other reasons for being than the promotion of health. Supporting the use of solitary confinement, he denied, as a medical expert, that it damaged the mind; but he also argued that if in some cases such damage ensued, the penal authorities were not necessarily to be blamed:

> Our system of separate confinement [he argued to the Carnarvon Committee] does not appear to affect the mind injuriously. I do not mean to say that a prisoner who comes into prison upon the verge of unsoundness of mind, might not develop into full unsoundness in that time, partly because of the separation; but I am of opinion also, that a prisoner should expect that that may happen to him, and that the possibility of unsoundness must be taken into account as one of the results of his being in prison at all; and that the possible falling into illness should be taken into account as the possible result of his being in prison at all; so also if he does those things which bring illness upon him, such illness being in no case the fault of those who have to deal with him, he ought to suffer for his own

> acts, and we should not be required to prevent him from making himself ill.[42]

Blending aspects of Farr and Chadwick, Guy joined two faces of Benthamism and of nineteenth-century public administration. He had a distinguished career of public service, advancing both scientific knowledge of the conditions of public and personal health, and advocating state action to apply this knowledge to eliminate remediable forms of ill health. Yet he was also a strong supporter of social discipline in general, and severe punishment of lawbreakers in particular. In his career and his outlook, as in that of many other persons who bridged the medical and the penal worlds of nineteenth-century Britain, the complex (but not thereby censurable) character of Utilitarian ideals was enacted.

This complex balance in Guy's career, which could be traced, in a minor key, in the careers of other prison medical officers, altered after his generation, as standards of what constituted proper 'care' steadily rose, and the acceptability of overt 'punishment' declined. The 1895 Gladstone Committee on Prisons began a process of reconstructing the presuppositions and practices of the penal system, and by the 1960s 'care' had presumably taken pride of place over 'punishment'. Yet, after criticism from the Left – both old (that, despite professions, there remained too little care, and too much punishment) and new (that care itself was really a more sinister form of punishment), and from the Right (that the trend of the twentieth century had been a mistake, and that punishment needed to be brought back), policy today appears to be in a muddle. It would appear that ideological simplifications from both Right and Left cannot abolish the tension Bentham perceived two centuries ago; what the former, somewhat disillusioned, director of the Massachusetts Prison Health Project, Curtis Prout, recently called a 'central irony' of penal policy: 'the same institution that is responsible for punishing offenders is also responsible for giving them the care they need'.[43] The experience of our nineteenth-century predecessors may still have much to teach us about living with this irony.

Notes

1. See Martin J. Wiener, 'The Unloved State: Twentieth-Century Politics in the Writing of Nineteenth-Century History', *Journal of British Studies*, July 1994.
2. M. J. Cullen, *The Statistical Movement in Early Victorian Britain* (Hassocks, Sussex: Harvester, 1975), 187.
3. Elie Halevy, *The Growth of Philosophic Radicalism* [first English

edition,1928](Boston: Beacon Press, 1955), 74.

4. L. J. Hume, 'Revisionism in Bentham Studies'. *Bentham Newsletter* no. 1 (May 1978), 3–20, and *Bentham and Bureaucracy* (Cambridge: Cambridge University Press, 1981).
5. *The Rationale of Punishment* (London, 1830), 354.
6. Gertrude Himmelfarb's brilliant 1965 essay, 'The Haunted House of Jeremy Bentham', revived awareness of Bentham's Panopticon scheme and paved the way for Michel Foucault's highly influential book, *Discipline and Punish.* However, both Himmelfarb and Foucault blurred the distinction between penal and general Benthamism, indicting Benthamism in general much too sweepingly, and also anachronistically exaggerated the totalitarianism even of penal Benthamism [see Janet Semple, 'Bentham's Haunted House', *Bentham Newsletter* no.11 (June 1987), 35–44, and 'Foucault and Bentham: A Defence of Panopticism', *Utilitas,* vol. 4, no. 1 (May 1992), 105–20].
7. *Political Economy* (1836), quoted in Walter Houghton, *The Victorian Frame of Mind 1830–1870* (New Haven, Conn.: Yale University Press, 1957), 249.
8. *The Works of Jeremy Bentham, published under the superintendence of his executor John Bowring* (Edinburgh: W. Tait, 1843) [hereafter called *Bowring*], vol. 4, 174.
9. *Introduction to the Principles of Morals and Legislation,* (ed.) J. H. Burns & H. L. A. Hart (London: Athlone Press, 1970), 158.
10. *Bowring,* vol. 4, 121.
11. *Bowring,* vol. 4, 123.
12. See Philip Priestley, *Victorian Prison Lives: English Prison Biography 1830–1914* (London: Methuen, 1985), and Joe Sim, *Medical Power in Prisons: The Prison Medical Service in England 1774–1989* (Milton Keynes: Open University Press, 1990).
13. In 1837, Farr had written Chadwick to urging him forward in his plans for a public health inquiry [13 Feb., 1837: University College London, Chadwick Papers [hereafter CP], file #714].
14. 'First Report of H. M. Commissioners Appointed to Inquire into the State of the Poor Laws in England and Wales 1834', Appendix A, Pt III.
15. Letter to Chadwick from D. Barry (an Irish prison official), 22 Dec., 1834: CP file #252.
16. Supported by 'hard-line' protégés like Charles Mott, a private contractor for the maintenance of paupers and lunatics under the Old Poor Law for whom Chadwick got an appointment as an assistant Poor Law Commissioner, and whom he later recommended for a prison governorship ('he would be pre-eminently successful in getting labour out of prisoners', he assured Sir Rowland Hill in 1842, since he had had much experience in dealing with 'refractory able-bodied paupers' [Chadwick to Hill, 31 Oct., 1842: CP file #1018]); Mott passed on the criticism even before Barry did, but disparaged it as not

altering Chadwick's thoroughly sound conclusions. Mott agreed with Chadwick on the need to guard against 'artful deceptions of the Paupers' who claimed to be sick [Mott to Chadwick, 11 Aug., 1834: CP file #1449].

17. See Anthony Brundage, *England's 'Prussian Minister': Edwin Chadwick and the Politics of Government Growth 1832–1854* (University Park, PA: Pennsylvania State University Press, 1988), 42, 48.
18. *Lancet*, 1837–8, I, 780. See Chadwick to Dr Laycock, 13 Apr., 1844: CP file #2181.
19. *Lancet*, 1837–8, I, 780.
20. *Ibid.*
21. For Farr's further criticisms of Chadwick in 1844, see John Eyler, *Victorian Social Medicine: The Ideas and Methods of William Farr* (Baltimore, MD: Johns Hopkins University Press, 1979), 70; for Chadwick's criticisms of Farr, see R. A. Lewis, *Edwin Chadwick and the Public Health Movement* (London: Longmans, Green, 1952), 32–3.
22. For all his expertise, Farr himself was not above dubious comparisons that supported his opinions: in an 1854 essay on 'Vital Statistics' he claimed that 'prisoners at the time of their committal must be considered in the same light as those who seek to assure their lives'; comparing the 12,886 persons between the ages of 20 and 40 who entered the Equitable Assurance Society in 1837 with prisoners committed in that year, he found mortality in the year following almost five times higher in the latter group [J. R. McCulloch, *A Statistical Account of the British Empire* (London: Longman; 4th edition, revised, 1854), II, 566].
23. For Farr prison conditions were simply one front in a general war on avoidable death of all sorts. In his annual reports from the General Registry Office Farr frequently criticized coroners' juries for their lack of thorough investigation of the causes of deaths, and their tendency to fall back on 'act of God' as all-purpose explanation.
24. In his anonymous critique of Chadwick's 1834 calculations, Farr had contemptuously noted that his chief motive seemed to be to minimize costs for his employers, the Poor Law Commissioners [op. cit.].
25. S. E. Finer, *The Life and Times of Sir Edwin Chadwick* (London: Methuen, 1952), 165, citing his unpublished manuscript for the Constabulary Commission Report of 1839: 'He maintained that because of the Howards and the Frys the prisons had been so reformed by "narrow sentiment and blind zeal" as actually to *attract* vagrants and others who preferred their comfort to labour. He put the excess cost of prisoners over their subsistence cost at more than £80,000 per annum.'
26. Chadwick to William Brebner, 26 Nov., 1841: CP file #365. By this time, Chadwick had come to see prisons as so healthy as to be models for general public health: one of the aims of his public health inquiry was 'to determine to what extent the health of the labouring classes might be increased if their habitations were made as cleanly and dry

and they were as well ventilated and warmed as the prison cells, if their diet were as regular and their persons as cleanly' [Chadwick to George Burgess, 29 Oct., 1841: CP file #407].

27. 'Vital Statistics', (note 22).
28. 1810–1885.
29. Sean McConville, *A History of English Prison Administration. Volume One: 1750–1877* (London: Routledge, 1981), 452. A formal position of Chief Medical Superintendant for the prison system as a whole was not created until 1878.
30. *Dictionary of National Biography*, vol. 8, 835.
31. On his death he was described as possessed of 'a mind of great breadth and a spirit of the purest philanthropy', *Lancet*, 1885, II, 554 (19 Sept., 1885).
32. William A. Guy, *Public Health: A Popular Introduction to Sanitary Science* (London, 1870), 216.
33. William A. Guy, 'John Howard's True Place in History', *Journal of the Statistical Society*, 38 (Dec. 1875), 430.
34. *Ibid.*, 435.
35. *Ibid.*, 437.
36. See Priestley, *op. cit.*, and Sim, *op. cit.*
37. The dietary, he warned, 'is not to my mind a satisfactory form of punishment' [Select Committee of the House of Lords on Gaol Discipline (Carnarvon Committee), *Parliamentary Papers*, 1863 (499), IX, 367].
38. *Ibid.*, 369.
39. The record at Millbank is ambivalent: despite his remarks to the Carnarvon Committee in 1863, after he assumed his post in 1859 dietary punishments per capita decreased for women but increased for men, slightly increasing overall [annual reports of the Directors of Convict Prisons].
40. William A. Guy, 'On Insanity and Crime; and on the Plea of Insanity in Criminal Cases', *Journal of the Statistical Society*, 32 (June 1869), 160.
41. William A. Guy, 'On Some Results of A Recent Census of the Population of the Convict Prisons in England', *Transactions of the National Association for the Promotion of Social Science 1863*, 569, 572, 574. He went on to note that 'it ought not to be forgotten, that the objects of all this watchful solicitude are not the mixed groups of debtors and criminals of every degree, on whose behalf John Howard exerted himself, but the most depraved, the most reckless, the most violent, the most brutal of mankind' (574).
42. *PP* 1863 (499), IX, 370.
43. Curtis Prout and Robert N. Ross, *Care and Punishment: The Dilemmas of Prison Medicine* (Pittsburgh, PA: University of Pittsburgh Press, 1988), 228.

4

Development of the Prison Medical Service, 1774–1895

Anne Hardy

In 1876, the celebrated medical humanitarian, Benjamin Ward Richardson, noted with some satisfaction that 'nothing in the sanitary history of this country is so astonishing as the history of gaols within 100 years'. The gaol, Richardson maintained, 'has been transformed into the most perfect of dwelling houses from the point of view of health.... Epidemic disease is under instant control. Disease from exposure to extremes of atmospheric variation, from impure air, excess, or want, from uncleanliness, personal or general, are out of the question. In a word, the occupant of the modern prison house is subject practically to none other than his acquired or inherited disease.'[1]

By 1876, the English prison had clearly come a long way from the typhus-haunted slums that so stirred the reforming instincts of eighteenth-century liberals like John Howard. And it is true that epidemic diseases had virtually disappeared from English prisons by 1850. This disappearance was largely a tribute to the efforts of lay reformers, and not to medical men.

Medical services to prisons were ramshackle until at least 1850. Although the Health of Prisoners Act 1774 provided for the appointment of prison surgeons, such appointments were optional, and were not made in many local prisons. In the 1820s, following reforms introduced by Sir Robert Peel when Home Secretary,[2] physicians or surgeons were appointed to most gaols, but such appointments were usually part-time, of local GPs with no special skills, who attended the prison only in emergencies, or at most for a couple of hours a day. It was only with the Prisons Act 1865 that medical appointments in prisons achieved a more regulated footing. Under this Act, which applied to local English prisons only, surgeons registered under the Medical Act 1858 were to be appointed, and they were given a distinct schedule of responsibilities, including the instruction to visit the prison twice a week at least, and to see each prisoner during that time.[3]

Historians give various dates for the emergence of the English Prison Medical Service. For Joe Sim, it begins with the Act of 1774, for Richard Smith with the incorporation of the local prison service under government control in 1877.[4] If, however, the prison medical service is considered as a professional entity, providing full-time careers for dedicated employees,[5] it is clear that the formation of the Prison Medical Service should be dated to 1850, when the passing of the Act for the Better Government of Convict Prisons (13 & 14 Vict c. 39) brought the convict prisons under central government control.

The character and ethos of the English prison service were changing in the decades around 1850.[6] The gradual ending of the transportation system led to the introduction of the new sentence of penal servitude, a minimum sentence of five years comprising initial periods of hard labour and separate confinement, followed by labour at public works. These sentences were worked out in special convict prisons, which the government began building in the 1840s. A two-tier structure of prison provision thus continued, despite the phasing out of transportation, with local prisons catering for short sentences, and convict prisons for long ones. By 1850, the convict prison service comprised five major prisons – Millbank, Pentonville, Portland, Parkhurst and Dartmoor (plus the prison hulks, soon to be abolished, and rented cells in county and borough gaols), and it was in these that a recognizable cadre of prison medical officers emerged.

The medical officers of the convict prisons quickly established themselves as a distinct professional group: they had common professional interests, served a common authority, participated in a recognizable career structure, and evolved for themselves a distinct professional ethos. The first officers were appointed to the convict prisons in the 1840s, and were men of experience. Several had formerly been naval surgeons; other, younger men had at least held one hospital post before entering the service. Once appointed into the prison service, however, they generally made a substantial part of their subsequent careers within it. Their posts were full-time and resident (except for that of the Superintendent at Millbank), and they usually had the help of an assistant surgeon. The assistant surgeons themselves often made their careers within the service, holding assistant posts in one or more prisons before being promoted to the dignity of medical officer.

The achievement of medical officer status did not necessarily mean a career spent within one prison. Although some medical officers, like

Charles Lawrence Bradley of Pentonville and J. D. Rendle of Brixton, followed such a path, many did not. As civil servants, skilled medical officers were often moved between prisons as the demands of the service required. Thus John Burns, after 25 years at Chatham, found himself supervising the medical arrangements at newly-opened Borstal in 1874. Dartmoor; meanwhile, functioned as a starting post for the careers of its medical officers between 1850 and 1870. Of five medical officers appointed there between 1852 and 1870, four moved on to other prisons, and one retired from the service because of ill health. Thus Vans Christian Clarke served at Dartmoor from 1863 to 1865, and then at Portsmouth and Pentonville before reaching what had been the pinnacle of the service, the appointment at Millbank, in 1878. Francis Askham, similarly, began as assistant surgeon under Clarke at Dartmoor before succeeding him in 1865. He subsequently served at Woking Female Prison, Portland and Portsmouth.

The convict prison service was at its apogee in the years between 1850 and 1885. By the mid-1880s, the sustained fall in the number of penal sentences had so reduced the convict population that a radical reorganization of the service was undertaken, and many convict prisons were closed.[7] Between 1882 and 1892, ten convict prisons with accommodation for more than 7,000 prisoners were assigned to other public purposes. Pentonville and Wormwood Scrubs, for example, were transferred to the local prison sector; Chatham was handed over to the Admiralty; Woking (Males and Females) to the War Office.[8] With the reduction in the number of convict prisons, and greater integration with the local prison service, the convict prison medical officers began to lose their distinctive identity. Some retired and left the service, others transferred into the local sector. George Walker, for example, was Medical Officer at Chatham until 1892; by 1893 he was Medical Officer at Holloway, where he remained until 1897 before becoming Governor and Medical Officer at Aylesbury Female Convict Prison, a position he held until his retirement in 1908.

The local prison service also experienced extensive reorganization after it was taken under central government control in 1877, with a reduction in the number of surgeons from 109 to 70 initially. Conditions in the local prison medical service remained rather different, however, with many officers continuing to serve part-time, but it is likely that the two types of service drew closer after 1877. Two new posts were established following the 1877 Act, that of Medical Inspector of Local Prisons, and that of Superintending Medical Officer of Convict Prisons. These were filled by the same man, suggesting that standards and methods in the two services are likely to have drawn closer together. Robert Gover, who filled these posts from their creation until his retirement in July 1896, had previously been Medical Officer of Millbank, and was highly respected both inside and outside the service. A gentle and unassuming man, invariably courteous and affable to his peers, he is known to have upheld the interests of prison medical staff, and to have been thoroughly involved in the reorganization of the local medical services after 1877.[9]

For most of the Victorian period, however, there were two branches of the prison medical service, with very different workloads and responsibilities, confronting different problems, managing different types of population, and responsible to different authorities. The wider history of the Prison Medical Service in this period is thus complex, and worthy of more extended treatment than can be attempted here. One question, however, is central to any historical discussion of the Prison Medical Service: was it the prisoner's friend, or was it the lackey of authority?[10]

The career of William Augustus Guy (1810–1885) provides a convenient vehicle for examining this question. Guy was Superintending Medical Officer at Millbank between 1859 and 1865. The Millbank post was the senior post in the service; since its opening as the first penitentiary in 1821, Millbank's physician had acted as unofficial adviser to the government on prison medical questions. Guy's predecessor, William Baly (1814–1861), had fulfilled this function admirably, and had made Millbank the focus of his career after his appointment in 1841 at the age of 27.[11] In this respect, Baly fitted snugly into the model of the convict prison medical officership as it developed after 1850. Guy was a very different kettle of fish. Unlike most other post-1850 appointees, he came to the convict service from outside. A fourth-generation medical man, with an established reputation as a sanitarian, he was already nearly fifty, and had been first Professor of Forensic Medicine and subsequently Dean of King's College, London since 1838. His motives for taking on the Millbank medical officership are obscure: perhaps he wanted to extend his forensic expertise by viewing criminals at closer quarters; perhaps he was tempted by the opportunity to make practical contributions to the prison system. Whatever his motive, he left the prison service in 1865, and returned to King's College as Professor of Hygiene. He continued, however, to act as an independent expert on prison medical questions until physical weakness got the better of him around 1880. It is perhaps significant that his position at Millbank is not mentioned in any of his obituaries, although his later service on the Royal Commission on Penal Servitude (1878) and the Departmental

Commission on Criminal Lunacy (1880–2) was.[12]

Guy came into the prison service not only with an established career behind him, but with firmly established social and political convictions. (His *Lancet* obituarist noted that his views on religion, politics and social science were 'far in advance of his time'.)[13] He was possessed of a peculiar brand of Benthamism, which abhorred waste, and saw idleness as the root of society's problems.[14] His ideas were perhaps most clearly articulated in the pamphlet *The Evils of England Social and Economic*, which he published in 1846, and are well expressed in the passage from Ecclesiasticus which he chose as its epigraph:

> Do well unto him that is lowly, but give it not unto the ungodly; hold back thy bread, and give it not unto him, lest he overmaster thee thereby.

Guy's central concern – like that of many in the 1840s – was the condition of England, but his solution to national crisis was an unusual one. He loathed what he called 'soup-kitchen philanthropy' ('that ingenious form of self-indulgence'), as much as he loathed 'Idleness, Drunkenness, Carelessness and Waste'.[15] He held that personal industry had made 'our glorious constitution' possible, and advocated starvation as a 'proper and expedient' punishment for idleness. He wished to achieve both economy and social justice: 'My blood boils within me', he confessed,[16]

> as I see the honest and hardworking English labourer, with an Irish rebel on one shoulder, an English pauper on the other, a dead weight of taxation on his back, and a crowd of beggars, thieves and vagrants pulling at his skirts and picking his pockets.

Guy was fully aware of the opprobrium his views were likely to attract, but was unrepentant: 'My apparent indifference to suffering', he told his readers, 'is that of the surgeon who performs a painful operation, that he may save the life of the patient.'[17] And pulling a further biblical justification out of his store, he recalled the 'sternly merciful precept of St Paul' – 'If any will not work, neither shall he eat'. The clarity and coherence with which Guy stated his case reinforced the strength of his views; his *Lancet* obituarist phrased it more discreetly: 'Work he held the natural remedy for human ills, and idleness their foster parent.'[18]

Guy's concern for the social and economic welfare of English society, and his unyielding views on the discipline required to achieve social justice, appear to have changed little during his later career and were reflected in his views on prison discipline and organization. His perspective on prison problems was essentially that of a layman, and was shaped by his established personal convictions. Within the Prison Medical Service, he was a maverick, an outsider whose independent status gave him standing with the disciplinary authorities, but whose views set him at odds with the prevailing ethos of the convict prison medical service. Guy's rigorous views and strong personality hardly qualified him as a lackey, but they certainly predetermined his reinforcement of the precepts of authority.

During the first twelve years of government control, the convict prisons were supervised by Sir Joshua Jebb, a humane and thoughtful man, who achieved significant improvements in the quality of prisoners' lives, and who willingly considered suggestions by governors and medical officers.[19] In 1862, however, following a series of robberies in London, and growing fears about criminals who could no longer be transported, a new and harsher disciplinary attitude among the ruling classes towards criminals found legislative expression.[20] Of special significance for the convict prisons was the Select Committee of the House of Lords into prison discipline, chaired by Lord Carnarvon. One of the central concerns of this Committee was prison diet and how to quantify, in Joe Sim's words, a just measure of pain to the nearest micro-ounce without compromising prison discipline.[21] Guy was a witness before the Committee, and his stern views on what should be the desirable features of a prison diet were very plain in his evidence. In particular, he recommended a uniform diet in prisons; deplored the inclusion of such items as treacle, molasses and cocoa; considered the existing first- and second-class prison diets too good; and was unable to agree with a previous witness (the physiologist Edward Smith) who declared that bread and water for a week was starvation.[22]

The Carnarvon Committee felt unable on its own account to reduce prison dietary, but recommended the appointment of a scientific committee of inquiry to establish a new dietary regime for the prisons. Much to the outrage of the *Lancet* this committee, when appointed, consisted not of 'scientific persons of experience, accustomed to physiological experiment' like William Sharpey, Edward Smith or Henry Acland, but of three prison medical officers: William Guy, Vans Christian Clarke (newly appointed at Dartmoor after an exciting naval career), and Dr Maitland of Gosport military prison.[23] (It should be noted, however, despite the *Lancet*'s claims, that the science of human nutrition was decidedly in its infancy at this time.)

The scientific committee's eventual recommendations were based on premises later set out by Guy for the information of the Royal Commission on Penal Servitude. First, to prevent scurvy by including potatoes and vegetables; second, to prevent diseases like scrofula and respiratory tuberculosis which might partly be attributed to insufficient nutrition; third, to ensure that the quantity of food was adjusted to the specific physical requirements of prisoners, depending on whether they were employed in sedentary occupations or on public works; and lastly, to set safe punishment diets.[24] As previous historians have pointed out, the aim of the committee was to achieve as spare a diet as would maintain the prisoner's health, without making any concessions that could be construed as a reduction in discipline.[25]

With this end in view, the committee eventually set a more varied diet by reducing the amount of meat and including some cheese and vegetables, but reduced the total amount of food given to the inmates of convict prisons. At Millbank, Pentonville, Brixton and Parkhurst, where convicts had physically relatively undemanding occupations, the weekly allowance of solid food was reduced from 306 ounces to 284; in the public works prisons it was reduced from 352 to 299 ounces, or by nearly one day's rations in the week.[26] A comparison of Guy's evidence before the Carnarvon Committee with the eventual outcome of the Committee of Scientific Inquiry suggests that he played a decisive part in formulating the recommendations.

The downwards revision of the food allowances brought the issue of diet squarely to the forefront of the convict prison medical officers' concerns. Until 1864, although the Home Office had a recommended dietary, this was not rigidly adhered to, and medical officers were allowed leeway in making alterations and extra allowances.[27] Under the new system, Guy's dietary was enforced in all the prisons (except the invalid prison at Woking) from 1864, and alterations and additions to the dietary were actively discouraged. For the most part the prisoners themselves seem to have accepted the new dietary quietly, although there was a mutiny at Portland, where the reductions were greatest, and much grumbling at Chatham.[28] The convict prison medical officers greeted the change cautiously: Guy and Clarke were – naturally – the only ones positively to approve the change in their annual reports.

By the following year, 1865, concern over the new dietary was beginning to manifest itself. William Houghton of Portland was asking for the reintroduction of tea at suppertime for his convicts, 'as was done formerly'. And he added, 'The new scale of diet I am inclined to think will not bear reduction; I would rather see some increase, particularly for those employed at hard labour.' Of the penal class prisoners, whose diet had also been reduced, he noted a loss of weight and the onset of 'obscure scorbutic symptoms'; the health of these prisoners declined more or less after three months on the diet, 'according to the strength of the individual'.[29] At Chatham in the same year, John Burns noted for the first time in print that his prisoners were suffering colic from eating tallow, refuse, and herbs found on the public works site.[30] In 1866, Burns became alarmed by a sharp deterioration in the health of known consumptives at Chatham, and managed to induce the Directors to grant a slight increase in diet. This, however, did not help the prisoners to gain weight, and was 'scarcely sufficient to make them effective for the labour of this place'.[31] (Convicts at Chatham were employed in building a sea-wall in the river, and were constantly in the wind and wet, digging mud from the river-bed.) In 1867, Burns reported that boils and carbuncles were more prevalent than formerly, and that he was dispatching prisoners suffering from debility to hospital, to recover their strength.[32] By 1868, Burns had negotiated extra diet for his consumptives, who were in addition carefully watched, and sent to the infirmary when necessary.[33]

Prisoners in the prison hospitals were allowed increased rations, which proved a great attraction to malingerers, but the prison hospital record also provides evidence for the inadequacy of Guy's diets. Although Valerie Johnston has rightly pointed out that prisoners' rations compared not unfavourably in many instances with the diets of ordinary labourers,[34] evidence from the public works prisons at least suggests that the balance between the two shifted after 1870. It is generally accepted among historians that rising living standards in the general population brought improved nutrition after 1870, and David Hamilton has argued that this was reflected in reduced rates of surgical mortality through increased resistance to wound infection.[35] However, nutritional status also has a significant bearing on the body's ability to heal, and in the convict prisons the 1864 dietary appears to have added complications to accident and surgical cases.

Victorian doctors were well aware of a relationship between health and healing. Already in 1857, William Houghton had noted that the convalescence of some accident cases was 'tedious, the bones not uniting readily'. This, he declared, was due to impaired health, and a generous diet was necessary, with 'wine and porter, tonic medicines, iron and quinine and lime water'.[36] Houghton was, however, proud of his surgical record. The convicts at Portland were engaged in stone quarrying, and accidents were frequent at the wagons and cranes during loading, and he often had to deal with compound and comminuted fractures, and extensive lacerated wounds. Yet he claimed to practise conservative surgery with great success: 'I have always adopted the conservative principles in surgery, and save all limbs, when possible from amputation. This is a mechanical operation and could be performed by any carpenter or butcher, but the beauty and science of surgery consists in preserving the limbs and rendering them of use to the patient.'[37] Houghton does not seem to have had serious problems with his surgical patients.

Ten years later, however, his successor, E. S. Blaker, was having problems, and poor nutrition was clearly implicated. 'Primary operations as a rule do very badly', Blaker recorded in 1870, 'fingers and toes very frequently require to be amputated, necrosis of the end bones ensues in fully one third of cases.' Significantly he added: 'If a man can be kept in hospital for a fortnight or three weeks before an operation, the wound almost always heals well. This I think points to the fact that the men as a body are below the normal standard of health.'[38] By 1871, Blaker had concluded that the 'total quantity of daily nourishment' was insufficient for men at hard labour.[39]

The observations of the convict prison medical officers were reinforced by increasing concern outside the prison service.[40] In 1869, for example, the *Lancet* observed that convicts were men whose constitutions were usually 'deteriorated by vice and privation, and whose physiques require therefore to be raised rather than lowered', adding tartly: 'We do not advocate the coddling of criminals; but, on the score of economy as well as humanity, it is wise to diminish the list of medical comforts by increasing the supply of butcher's meat.' [41]

Goaded by this accumulating criticism, the Directors of Convict Prisons arranged for an inquiry into the sufficiency of the diet in 1872. The man whom they appointed to conduct it was William Guy. Not surprisingly, considering that he had designed the dietary in the first place, Guy found that none of the opinions critical of the dietary rested on any firm basis of fact.[42] Indeed the determination of the non-medical authorities to maintain the disciplinary diet is clearly demonstrated by their continued use of Guy in such investigations. Having retired from Millbank in 1865, Guy as Professor of Hygiene at King's College bore all the appearance of an independent authority in his continuing association with prison questions in the later 1860s and 1870s. He was one of the two medical experts appointed to the Royal Commission on Penal Servitude of 1878; the other was Headlam Greenhow, a distinguished sanitarian, who had been on the Royal Commission which inquired into the treatment of treason-felony prisoners in 1870. As a member of that Commission, Greenhow had approved Guy's dietary.[43] It therefore comes as no surprise that the 1878 Penal Servitude Commission reiterated approval of the 1864 dietary, concluding firmly that 'prison diet ought in all cases to be strictly limited to what is necessary to maintain prisoners in health, and to enable them to perform the work imposed upon them'.[44]

Not surprisingly either, none of these affirmations convinced the prison medical officers, although they did reduce the amount of explicit criticism they indulged in. But they also developed strategies to resolve the problems which insufficient diet created. The chief of these was the hospitalization of men suffering from 'debility' until they were sufficiently restored to return to work. In 1872, 245 prisoners were so treated at Chatham; in 1886–7, 355 were similarly restored at Portland. Such numbers were representative in a policy which continued into the 1890s.[45]

Guy's determined adherence to a stern disciplinary diet despite criticism on medical grounds from both within and without the prison service gives a good indication of his general stand in prison matters. In outlook and sympathy he was much closer to the non-medical, non-prison service people who determined disciplinary policy from a lay perspective than he was to the constructive civil service approach of his medical colleagues in the convict service. The attitude of the latter to lay authority was in many respects similar to that of the doctors who worked for the local authorities and the Poor Law Board: they tried to accommodate what they perceived to be the needs of their 'clients' – whether prisoners, the sick poor or the general public – within the constraints imposed by the system within which they worked. Just as medical officers in the Poor Law Board's infectious disease hospitals admitted non-pauper cases at their own discretion,[46] so the convict medical officers used their discretion to transfer starving men to hospital.

The difference between Guy and most of the prison medical officers was again illustrated by the issue of hard labour, first class; that is, the use of the treadmill and other instruments of unproductive punishment labour. The first month of a sentence of penal servitude was spent in this unrelenting regime of pointless disciplinary punishment, and sentences of hard labour, first class were also served in the local prisons. The system was widely, though not universally, disliked within both local and convict prison services.[47] The Carnarvon Committee, which approved the use of the treadmill, and recommended that it be used more extensively, none the less found only one witness wholeheartedly in its favour – Sir Walter Crofton, superintendent of the Irish prisons.[48] Guy, also a witness, was not called upon to express an opinion after he admitted that although Millbank possessed a treadmill, it was never used.[49]

Following the incorporation of the local prisons under central government supervision in 1877, however, the disciplinary objective of uniformity of practice in all aspects of the prison system led to a review of hard labour practice in the local prisons. This review was undertaken by Robert Gover, Guy's successor at Millbank, who had just been appointed Medical Inspector of the local prisons. Gover, in contrast to Guy, was very much the professional prison medical officer. He spent the whole of his career in the prison service, beginning as assistant surgeon at Portsmouth in 1857, rising to be resident surgeon at Millbank under Guy, and finally succeeding him as Superintending Medical Officer there in 1865. As previously noted, he was in public a gentle and courteous man; his approach to his work was thoughtful and pragmatic; and he had the distinction of being spoken of with unqualified approval by the ex-convict Henry Harcourt, an otherwise bitter critic of prison medical officers, before the 1878 Commission. In Harcourt's opinion, 'a more humane and better man does not exist than Dr Gover'.[50]

Gover's report on hard labour has been cited by previous historians, and has generally been construed as approving the use of the treadmill.[51] In fact the case was otherwise, and the story reflects the continuing tension between the disciplinary ethos of the administrative authorities on the one hand, and medical recognition of the undesirability of this type of labour on the other. Convict medical officers in general tacitly deplored the treadmill. They constantly noted the poor condition of men received from the county and borough gaols (although this also reflected on the dietaries of those prisons), and in 1870 Vans Clarke went so far as to comment on the 'spectre-like attenuation' of prisoners received after treadmill labour.[52] Although disapproval of the treadmill was usually couched in terms of the psychological effects of 'unproductive' labour on the morale and behaviour of prisoners,[53] the physical effects of this relentless form of mindless punishment did not go unobserved. By 1895, when Guy had been dead for ten years, all classes of witness before the Gladstone Committee were agreed that as an occupation, the treadmil lwas 'most undesirable'.[54]

In 1878, however, abolition of the treadmill was not on the cards. Gover's task was to review the practice of hard labour in local prisons, and to recommend ways of making practice uniform. On one level Gover did indeed express approval of the treadmill, but, significantly, only as the best available means for ensuring that the work, or punishment, was equitably distributed between the men engaged on it.[55] In fact, Gover's report suggests that he may even have considered the possibility of doing away with unproductive labour. He recorded having scrutinized the relevant legislation – the Prison Acts of 1865 and 1877 – very carefully, and noted his conclusion that the intention behind the definition of hard labour was very clear: a specific category of penal and deterrent labour was desired, and the treadmill, the shot-drill, the capstan and the crank were so strongly differentiated from other types of prison labour as to constitute such a category. It is hard not to hear a measure of disapproval in the observation that followed:[56]

> The legislators who framed these Acts would seem to have taken every precaution that occurred to them to ensure that every male prisoner sentenced to hard labour should be employed upon this repugnant description of work during at least a portion of his sentence.

If Gover had been considering recommending the abolition of this type of labour, the legislative provisions offered him no way out.

Gover's enquiries revealed that the daily treadmill task varied greatly between the different local prisons, from a daily minimum of 7,200 feet at Morpeth to 12,852 feet at Northallerton. His own recommendation was to standardize the task at 8,640 feet daily.[57]

The Prison Commissioners referred Gover's report to two outside experts, William Guy and G. W. Hastings,[58] who made mincemeat of Gover's concerns. They were highly critical of his attempt to secure an equitable distribution of labour between men on the treadmill. 'We conclude', they observed, 'that hard labour of the first class must necessarily be administered more or less in the rough.'[59] In other words, any concern for equity between prisoners was mere sentimentalism. Further, Guy and Hastings had no intention of endorsing Gover's recommendation of a relatively modest daily task – they thought it 'too low'. They made special enquiries, and could not discover that the task in use at Northallerton had resulted in any mischief or injury to prisoners. They recommended the adoption of 10,000 feet a day as the uniform task, with the rider that 'We are by no means certain that the amount of labour enforced at Northallerton would be excessive if generally adopted.'[60] However, even the Prison Commissioners' nerve failed here: they set a task of 9,000 feet daily, 'for the present, at least, to be on the safe side'. And in deference, evidently, to Gover's concern, they indicated a need to establish lower grades of task to suit prisoners who were not competent to perform the whole.[61]

As regards the bodily health of prisoners, Guy's influence on the later Victorian prison system can be seen to have been negative, and at some variance with the concerns of the professional convict prison medical officers who were, in the final event, responsible for the long-term welfare of prison inmates. While Guy's disciplinary rigour derived from his pre-existing convictions, and although extreme is comprehensible in the context of early Victorian criminal policy as described by Wiener, personal professional experience was a powerful determinant of professional attitudes within the Prison Medical Service. The importance of this experience is suggested not only by the convict prison medical officers' generally determined defence of prisoners' physical welfare, but also by their attitude towards insane and weak-minded prisoners, a subject on which, by the 1880s, they had come to share considerable common ground with Guy.

Insanity existed as a problem within the convict prison medical service from its beginnings in the 1840s. In the early years, concern focused on the effects of separate confinement, and whether or not it contributed to inducing or aggravating mental problems in prisoners.[62] Guy's predecessor at Millbank, William Baly, had been convinced that, in the long term, separate confinement did indeed pose a risk to sanity – especially for men 'of any considerable degree of imbecility, or great dulness of intellect', who would 'with certainty be rendered actually insane or idiotic by a few months' separate confinement'.[63] Many men of impaired or deficient mind were received into Millbank, he noted, and an increase in the number of truly insane was only prevented by transferring such men into association as soon as their condition became apparent to the medical officer.

Alongside the question of separate confinement, therefore, there already existed in the 1850s a recognized category of weak-minded persons coming into the prisons, which was causing the prison authorities concern. This concern increased steadily as the century advanced. Although John Campbell, Medical Officer of the Invalid Depot, then at Dartmoor, noted in 1852 that until very recently very few mental cases had come to his notice, he had charge of more than 80 weak-minded prisoners by 1855.[64] Campbell was anxious that such prisoners should be separated from the rest – although many were harmless, others were subject to fits of excitement, some constantly misbehaved themselves, and as a group they were a constant source of anxiety – and in 1856 an effective segregation of the weak-minded from the mentally fit was sanctioned.[65] Meanwhile the number of weak-minded prisoners continued to grow: by 1860 there were 126 of them at Dartmoor.

During the 1860s, Millbank functioned as an assessment centre for prisoners in questionable physical or mental health from both local and convict prisons. In his capacity as Superintending Medical Officer, William Guy thus came into contact with many such cases, and was, indeed, responsible for their assessment with such expert outside help as he deemed necessary.[66] There can be little doubt that Guy's prison experience aroused, or encouraged, his interest in the weak-minded as a social and criminal problem. One of the objects of the prison census, which he engineered in 1862, was to obtain information on the mental health of prisoners and its relation to the crimes committed.[67] Once tabulated, the information obtained proved to be in 'striking conformity' with the views which Guy, in his own words, 'should have been led to form by *a priori* reasoning, no less than by casual observation of prisoners'[68] – a phraseology which suggests (or perhaps was meant to suggest) that he came to the statistical information without preconceived ideas. Whether this was the case or not (*The Evils of England* says nothing about lunatics), he rapidly developed some. The statistics led him to infer that[69] 'weak-minded, insane and epileptic prisoners of both sexes, are especially addicted to the crime of arson; and also . . . to crimes consisting in or accompanied by violence; and that male prisoners answering to the same description are prone to the commission of a class of crimes often, but not always marked by violence. I speak of rape and offences *contra naturam.*'

Perhaps to further his observations, Guy arranged for the transfer of the weak-minded prisoners from Dartmoor to Millbank, where they remained as a special category until transferred again, to Parkhurst, in 1869.

Guy baled out of the Prison Medical Service in 1865, and returned to King's College; but the problem of the weak-minded prisoner continued to escalate, not only as a perceived problem within the convict prison medical service, but also within Guy's personal cosmology. By the time he was appointed to the Commission on Criminal Lunacy, at the age of seventy, the weak-minded had come to represent to him a very dangerous social evil. As a class, he wrote in a memorandum to his colleagues on the Commission,[70]

> They have very imperfect and indistinct ideas of the requirements of law, of legal proceedings, and of punishment ... they have strong passions and weak self-control; are easily led into temptation and participation in criminal acts by persons of stronger wills and characters than their own; they are much addicted to wandering from place to place, and apt to be dangerously impressed by topics which excite the public mind; they take a strange delight in fire raising and

> other malicious destruction of property, and go beyond persons afflicted with other forms of unsound mind in the commission of such offences as murder, arson, rape, and various forms of unnatural offence.

Guy's paranoia was not, however, confined to any recognized class of weak-minded persons, such as village idiots or such as recognizably might be confined to asylums; his fears had an apocalyptic dimension. 'There is', he continued,

> every reason to believe that these persons constitute an important section, if not a large majority, of the beggars, thieves, mendicant thieves, tramps, and vagabonds who infest our thoroughfares and fill the minds of the weaker and more helpless members of our society with constant apprehension. There can be no greater or more perilous mistake than to characterise such persons as harmless imbeciles.

Guy's opinion of imbeciles represents one extreme of a wide spectrum of concern with the weak-minded which existed both inside and outside the convict prison system by the 1880s.[71] At the heart of this concern lay the question of who was to have long-term custody of criminal lunatics and the criminal weak-minded. Neither the asylums nor the prisons wanted the responsibility,[72] and their representatives before the Criminal Lunacy Commission stressed the danger constituted by these classes to society. Dr Orange of Broadmoor, in response to leading questions posed by Guy, agreed that lunatics and imbeciles were alike dangerous, while Gover declared explicitly that 'criminal imbeciles are the most treacherous and dangerous set of men you can imagine; they are never harmless'.[73]

Behind these anxieties lay a joint prison and asylum experience of assaults by criminal lunatics on both inmates and staff. Orange's predecessor had had to retire following a serious assault by a Broadmoor inmate; while the abandoning of the Millbank assessment system in 1881 had unsatisfactory repercussions across the convict prison service. Thus in 1882, the Medical Officer for Brixton Prison noted that he did not have enough cell accommodation for troublesome mental cases, and no means of coping with them: 'I am completely at the mercy of these men', he noted.[74] At Woking, where most criminals of this type were housed between 1860 and 1891, there was a continuous record of serious assaults; in 1878, for example, there were 26 assaults on prison staff, most of which occurred when officers intervened in prisoner disputes. The prisoners tended to reserve their most serious assaults for each other: thus Reg. B. 1401 stabbed Reg. W. 321 in the loins, wounding him in the kidney, while Reg. C. 1341 bit an ear off Reg. C. 1478.[75] Such experiences inevitably coloured the views of prison medical officers obliged to deal with criminal lunatics. Arthur Mitchell, Guy's fellow medical on the 1882 Commission, acknowledged as much, noting that Guy's only experience was of prison imbeciles, and that he had therefore met and studied the very worst of them, who were but a handful of the whole body.[76]

Arthur Mitchell's experience of the weak-minded was diametrically opposed to that of the English prison medical officers. He had been employed by the Scottish Lunacy Board since its creation in 1857, was appointed Commissioner in Lunacy in 1870, and had been involved since its inception in the Scottish policy of caring for imbeciles in the community. The author of an influential manual entitled *The Insane in Private Dwellings*, he was a persuasive advocate of more sympathetic methods of treating the insane.[77] Mitchell's Scottish experience of managing the weak-minded in the community, and his practical, cogently expressed views on the care and control of the weak-minded put a balanced perspective on Guy's alarmism. The 1882 Commission's final outcome was clearly influenced by Mitchell's experience rather than by Guy's vision of hordes of vagrant imbeciles overturning the social order: the Commissioners recognized the unexpected extent and complexity of the social problem posed by the weak-minded, but found themselves unable to make recommendations, except for the possible future appointment of a specific commission to address the problem.[78]

Guy himself, however, remained unconvinced by Mitchell's very different perspective. In an essay published in 1884, the year before his death, he re-argued the case he had made before the Criminal Lunacy Commission, urging that imbeciles were 'pre-eminently dangerous' members of society who should be incarcerated for life, and that a body of mounted police should be constantly employed on the main roads to arrest all tramps and vagrants, who would then have their mental condition assessed before being consigned either to an asylum or the workhouse. 'May that good time come and soon', he concluded,[79]

> when our streets and thoroughfares being cleared of their dangerous classes, the poor rightly so called shall resume their right to be left alone, and the nation growing richer, one class with another, by the increase of money … the most ignorant and reckless of stump-orators shall not dare to set wealth and poverty in any way against each other.

There is an element of an old man's tragedy in this obsession of Guy's closing years, and more than a suggestion of the overriding preoccupation of his life: the battle he was fighting was still that for the condition of England, but his vision of the evils of England had extended beyond the mere idle, drunk and Irish, to encompass all these in the mentally deficient.

Yet if personal professional experience was crucial in forging the attitude of convict prison medical staff towards the weak-minded and insane, and if it forged in both Guy and Gover a deep-seated conviction of the dangerous character of such unfortunates, this personal experience also determined the differences in their attitudes towards the treatment of the sane able-bodied prisoner. In this respect it is tempting to contrast Guy's and Gover's approach to diet and treadmill labour, to draw attention to Guy the outsider's avid authoritarianism on the one hand and Gover the professional's tempered humanitarianism on the other. The contrast should not, however, be stretched too far. It was the prison medical officer's duty and responsibility to return fit men to society at the end of their prison sentences. Medical officers were perfectly aware of public criticism; of the damaging publicity generated by shattered constitutions and deaths in custody; of the consequences of treadmill labour and inadequate diet for men who too often brought the infection of tuberculosis or the potential for disablement through heart disease with them into prison.[80] Every tighter twist of the punishment screw dictated by the outraged morality of the legislature added to the pressures on them and raised the levels of stress inherent in their position. The Victorian medical profession was an overcrowded one, and prison medical officerships at least offered a secure income. But prison medical officers paid a price: they were at the centre of the tension between punishment and care which lay at the heart of the Victorian prison system.[81] 'Another year of anxious work has passed', wrote the Medical Officer for Dartmoor in 1878,[82]

> How anxious, none but a prison surgeon can fully comprehend. Unlike his confreres in the public hospitals he bears an undivided responsibility together with professional work of the most varied character … in addition to his hospital work he has in his charge everything relating to health in the prison so that ventilation, dietary, clothing, work, punishment, are all guided by him, the latter especially gives him much thought and anxiety; careful as he must be to make the convicts' health his first charge, and yet, at the same time not to screen the offender, or seem to interfere with the duties and prorogations of the discipline authority.

The stresses and anxieties inherent in the prison medical officers' extensive responsibilities came to a head over the thorny problem of malingering. Malingering was very much a part of prison culture in the 1870s and 1880s, with prisoners not only seeking by such means as lay within their power to avoid the terrible exertions of hard labour, but also to enjoy the enhanced peer-group status which successful malingering conferred.[83] The epidemic of factitious ulcers (induced by placing pieces of lime in boots, or by introducing thread or splinters beneath the skin and covering the part with lime) which spread from Portsmouth to Portland and Chatham in the late 1860s illustrates the scale of the problem: at Chatham alone in 1871, the number of ulcer cases increased from 98 in the previous year to 247.[84] Medical officers in these years were often significantly overworked and although the introduction of separate infirmary cells in prison hospitals after 1870 did something to reduce malingering, there were multiple roots to the problem. Thus Blaker noted in 1871 that the hospital had become less popular with the prisoners at Portland: 'One great proof of this is that malingering has wonderfully diminished of late.' He had all but given up prescribing alcohol and had replaced it by milk and beef-tea: 'doing my patients quite as much good, but not pleasing them equally well'.[85] Simple changes in the type of treatment offered could be more effective in reducing the attractions of a sick-bed than more draconian deterrents.

The frequency of malingering had more serious consequences than the overworking of medical officers in these decades: it helped to establish vicious circles of conflict between some prisoners and their medical superintendents. Evidence before the 1878 Royal Commission, notably that of the ex-convict Harcourt and of the Medical Officer Francis Askham, demonstrated that medical officers could and did react with brutal repression to persistent malingering. Convict prison medical officers were not uniformly benevolent, and the conditions of their employment and responsibility were such as both to aggravate personal tensions and to provide opportunities for their release. Yet such situations were created as much by individual circumstances as by the stress inherent to life in convict prisons. William Guy was one of the rare prison medical officers who rated society's requirements for punishment and discipline above convict health. He could afford to do so, for he was only briefly responsible for the health and safety of prisoners in any direct way. While force of circumstance and personal experience served to tip some convict prison medical officers into regimes of repressive brutality, the history of Guy's involvement with the Victorian Prison Medical Service demonstrates that many, perhaps most, prison medical officers valued their charges 'health, and were prepared not only to be critical of the values of authority, but to circumvent by such means as lay within their power, disciplinary instructions which they considered to be damaging to health.

Notes

1. Quoted in the Report of the Directors of Convict Prisons (RDCP) for 1876, *PP* 1877 xlv, 10.
2. Peel's Gaol Act, 4 George IV, c. 64, makes no specific provision for the appointment of surgeons, but the expectation of such an appointment is clear in section x of the Act.
3. Prisons Act 1865, 28 & 29 Vict c. 126, sec. 10; schedule 1, secs 86–92.
4. Joe Sim, 'Medical Power in Prisons', *The English Prison Medical Service 1774–1980* (Milton Keynes: Open University Press, 1990); Richard Smith, 'History of the prison medical service', *British Medical Journal*, 287 (1983), 1787.
5. On the structure and emergence of professional groups in this period see Harold Perkin, *The Rise of Professional Society, 1850–1950* (London: Routledge, 1990).
6. See Sean McConville, *A History of English Prison Administration. Volume One: 1750–1877* (London: Routledge and Kegan Paul, 1981), chapter 6 *et seq*.; Martin Wiener, *Reconstructing the Criminal. Culture, Law, and Policy in England, 1830–1914* (Cambridge: Cambridge University Press, 1990), chapters 1, 2; Janet Semple, *Bentham's Prison* (Oxford: Oxford University Press), 1993.
7. Wiener, *Reconstructing the Criminal*, chapter 7 *et seq*. For the social background to this transformation see Brian Harrison, *Peaceable Kingdom* (Oxford: Oxford University Press, 1982); F. M. L. Thompson, *The Rise of Respectable Society 1830–1900* (London: Fontana Paperbacks, 1988).
8. RDCP (1892–3), *PP* 1893–4 xlvii, 435.
9. *Lancet*, 1897, ii, 1644.
10. See above, Roy Porter, 'Howard's Beginning'. This question also runs through the discussions in Sim's *Medical Power in Prisons*, and Wiener's *Reconstructing the Criminal*.
11. *Lancet*, 1862, i, 147. Baly retired from Millbank when he was, to his own considerable surprise, made physician to Queen Victoria in 1859.
12. *Ibid*., 1885, ii, 554; *British Medical Journal*, 1885, ii, 573; *Dictionary of National Biography*.
13. *Lancet*, 1885, ii, 554.
14. For Guy as a Benthamite, see above, Martin Wiener, 'The Health of Prisoners'.
15. W. A. Guy, *The Evils of England Social and Economic* (London: John

W. Parker, 1846), 14–15.

16. *Ibid.*, 10.
17. *Ibid.*, 4. For the early Victorian view of pain as a necessary element to transformation, and the association between penal and medical discourse see Wiener, *Reconstructing the Criminal*, 111–23.
18. *Lancet*, 1885, ii, 554.
19. See, for example, RDCP *PP* 1854 xxxiii, 16–20.
20. J. E. Thomas, *The English Prison Officer since 1850. A study in conflict* (London: Routledge and Kegan Paul, 1972), 18.
21. Sim, *Medical Power*, p. 34. See also Michael Ignatieff, *A Just Measure of Pain: The Penitentiary in the Industrial Revolution, 1750–1850* (London: Macmillan, 1978).
22. Select Committee on the Present State of Discipline in Gaols and Houses of Correction (SCDG), *PP* 1863 ix, qq. 3804–3884. For Guy's stern attitude to diet see Valerie Johnston, 'Diet in workhouses and prisons, 1835–1895', unpublished D.Phil. thesis, Oxford University, 1981, 115–16.
23. *Lancet*, 1864, i, 675.
24. Royal Commission on the Penal Servitude Acts (RCPS), *PP* 1878–9, xxxvii, 36–7.
25. Sim, *Medical Power*, 34–5.
26. RDCP (1863), *PP* 1864 xxvi, 217.
27. See Johnston, 'Diet', pp. 106–7.
28. RDCP (1864), *PP* 1865 xxv, 11, 17, 168.
29. RDCP (1865), *PP* 1866 xxxviii, 111–12.
30. *Ibid.*, 141.
31. RDCP (1866), *PP* 1866 xxxvi, 174.
32. RDCP (1867), *PP* 1867–8 xxxiv, 738.
33. RDCP (1868), *PP* 1868–9 xxx, 257.
34. Johnston, 'Diet', 17–18.
35. David Hamilton, 'The nineteenth-century surgical revolution – antisepsis or better nutrition?', *Bulletin of the History of Medicine*, lvi (1982), 30–40.
36. RDCP (1857), *PP* 1857–8 xxix, 625.
37. RDCP (1859), *PP* 1860 xxxv, 567; see also *ibid.*, (1860), *PP* 1861 xxx, 445.
38. RDCP (1870), *PP* 1871 xxx, 218.
39. RDCP (1871), *PP* 1872 xxxi, 593.
40. Sim, *Medical Power*, 35–8.
41. *Lancet*, 1868, i, 441.
42. RDCP (1872), *PP* 1873 xxiv, 8–9.
43. RCPS, *PP* 1878–9 xxxvii, 38.
44. *Ibid.*
45. RDCP (1872), *PP* 1873 xxxiv, 330; *ibid.* (1886–7), *PP* 1887 xli, 834; *ibid.* (1894–5), *PP* 1895 lvi, 1279.
46. On the activities of medical staff in the infectious disease hospitals see

Gwendolen Ayers, *England's First State Hospitals* (London: Wellcome Trust, 1965), 61–2.

47. SCDG, *PP* 1863 ix, 573; *ibid.*, Appendix N, 505–6.
48. *Ibid.*, 574.
49. *Ibid.*, q. 3835.
50. RCPS, *PP* 1878–9 xxxvii, q. 4257.
51. Philip Priestley, *Victorian Prison Lives* (London: Methuen, 1985), 129; Sim, *Medical Power*, 43; Wiener, *Reconstructing the Criminal*, 128.
52. RDCP (1870), *PP* 1871 xxx, 58.
53. See, for example, SCDG (1863), qq 576–789, 2152–3.
54. Report of the Departmental Committee on Prisons, 1895 lvi, 23.
55. Report of the Commissioners of Prisons (1878) (RCP) , *PP* 1878–9 xxxiv, Appendix 15, 55.
56. *Ibid.*, 53.
57. *Ibid.*
58. George Woodyatt Hastings, barrister; son of Sir Charles Hastings, founder of the British Medical Association. He was General Secretary of the National Association for the Promotion of Social Science, and was elected MP for East Worcestershire in 1880. For the NAPSS see Laurence Goldman, 'The Social Science Association, 1857–1886: a context for mid-Victorian Liberalism', *English Historical Review*, 1986 (101), 95–134.
59. RCP (1878), *PP* 1878–9 xxxiv, Appendix 16, 65.
60. *Ibid.*
61. *Ibid.*, 11.
62. See Report on the Discipline and Management of Convict Prisons, *PP* 1852–3, li, 21–5, 118–27.
63. *Ibid.*, 23–5.
64. RDCP (1852), *PP* 1852–3, li, 595; *ibid.*, 1855, *PP* 1856 xxxv, 184.
65. RDCP (1856), *PP* 1857 session 2, xxiii, 326.
66. In 1860, for example, he called in the distinguished alienist Forbes Winslow to assist in evaluating a case: RDCP (1860), *PP* 1861 xxx, 237.
67. For his report on the census, see William Guy, 'On some results of a recent census of the population of the convict prisons in England', *Transactions of the National Association for the Promotion of Social Science* (TNAPSS), 1862, 561–80.
68. *Ibid.*, 565.
69. *Ibid.*, 564.
70. Commission on Criminal Lunacy (CCL), *PP* 1882 xxxii, Appendix B no. 1, 1002.
71. Wiener, *Reconstructing the Criminal*, 317–21; see also Andrew Scull, '*Museums of Madness* revisited', *Social History of Medicine*, 6 (1993), 20–2.
72. *Ibid.*, 320.

73. CCL, qq. 533–6 (Orange), 820 (Gover).
74. RDCP (1881–2), *PP* 1882 xxxiv, 64.
75. RDCP (1878), *PP* 1878–9 xxxv, 503–4.
76. CCL, Appendix B no. 2, 1006.
77. 'Sir Arthur Mitchell', *Dictionary of National Biography*, Supplement, 1901–1911, vol. II, 623.
78. CCL, 52–3.
79. W. A. Guy, *In the Footsteps of Count Rumford* (London: Harrison and Sons, 1884), 13.
80. See, for example, RDCP (1868), *PP* 1868–9 xxx, 333.
81. See Wiener, above, 44–59.
82. RDCP (1878), *PP* 1878–9 xxxv, 177, see also *ibid.*, (1883), *PP* 1884 xliii, 102.
83. RDCP (1868), *PP* 1868–9 xxx, 149.
84. *Ibid.*, *PP* 1872 xxxi, 687.
85. *Ibid.*, (1871), *PP* 1872 xxxi, 593.

Commentary

Hardy (In response to a question) The directors of convict prisons considered that penal sentences were having a deterrent effect, and that was why fewer convicts were coming to the jail.

Speaker You mentioned the report of the 1878–79 Commission. Could you comment on the evidence through that Commission which suggested that some prison medical officers were involved in systematic brutality?

Hardy I think that there was one prison medical officer in particular who was implicated and that is Henry Francis Askham. I am pretty sure that Askham was an unsatisfactory character, and he goes out of the Prison Medical Service almost immediately after that Commission. Not all of them were prisoners' friends: and cases of systematic brutality did occur.

Hardy (In response to a question) Increasingly after about 1860 mental problems were shuffled in the Prison Medical Service: they set up Woking Prison and Broadmoor as special institutions for housing mental cases and it is not something that really crosses the path to any great extent for the normal run of prison medical officers because as soon as somebody is showing signs of mental instability they are sent to Millbank for assessment and from there transferred to Woking.

Jean Loudon There is an absence of obituary mention of medical officers of the Millbank Penitentiary. Before 1850 there are plenty of obituary mentions of medical men who were also the local jail medical officers, including at least one who died of jail fever.

Hardy I think that what happens is that there is a change in the nature of the obituaries in the medical journals. As they become more interested in medicine and in medical research and in professional status, the journals lose interest in convict doctors and probably in local prison medical officers as well, because these people do not contribute to medical research and advancement. Gover is the only one among these I have been looking at, for whom there is an obituary (in the *Lancet* – there is none in the *British Medical Journal*). And it does actually suggest that in spite of the fact that nobody would have heard of him, because he had never done any research and never published anything outside his prison work, he nonetheless did deserve a small obituary. But there are several people who were really quite interesting in the Prison Medical Service: one of whom went on subsequently – Dr Brain – to be the medical officer at Broadmoor, and I have been unable to find an obituary in the medical press. Full-time prison medical officers were civil servants and do not generally merit an obituary notice. You find the same thing in medical officers of health, and in Poor-Law medical officers, even quite eminent ones, but they do not get obituaries, or where they do it is because they have done other things that make them interesting to the profession. Edwin Lancaster was a great coroner and his obituaries ignore the fact that he was medical officer of health for 10 years, and go on about his work as a coroner: and you find that pattern repeated.

Smith I can't give you the criteria which my forebears used for obituaries in the last century, but what I have to tell you is that obituaries are a complete nightmare for me because we obituarise everybody who gets their notice submitted in time: it's different with the *Lancet* which does what I would like to do, but cannot.

5

Elizabeth Fry and Mid-Nineteenth Century Reform

Anne Summers

Elizabeth Fry has entered the literature on prison reform more as an icon than as an historical figure whose activities are open to discussion and critical assessment. Those areas in which her labours were not crowned with success have either been discreetly ignored, or – in an inversion, rather than subversion of the traditional hagiography – treated as evidence of an idol's feet of clay.[1] In this essay it will be argued that Elizabeth Fry made a distinctive contribution to debates on the mental health of prisoners which was no less historically significant for going largely against the grain of official developments in penal discipline. It will also be suggested that Fry's contribution to the discussion of the health of prisoners in the widest sense was limited both by her own emphasis on the priority of moral regeneration, and by the restrictions placed by the authorities on the activities of lady prison visitors.

The nature of the sources used for this study dictates the provisional character of some of its conclusions. The 46 volumes of Elizabeth Fry's diary are largely concerned with spiritual and family matters. The only records apparently surviving of the British Ladies' Society for Promoting the Reformation of Female Prisoners (to be called hereafter the British Society) are two books of minutes, from which many pages have been removed, and which leave the last decade of her life practically unaccounted for. These materials, together with her family correspondence, a small number of publications on prison work, and her evidence to Parliamentary inquiries, enable us to gain at least a partial perspective on a reforming agenda that evolved over time and in collaboration with many other historical actors, known and unknown. But close local studies might fill many of the gaps, and turn negatives into positives. For the moment there remain, for the medical historian, frustrating discrepancies between the rich documentation in the diaries and family letters of a constant practical concern with the care and treatment of everyday illness, and the lack of similar references in her writings on sickness among prisoners.

Although the narrative of Elizabeth Fry's prison reforms is a familiar one, I shall recapitulate it briefly here. She first visited Newgate prison in early 1813, having been urged to do so by the American Quaker, Stephen Grellet, and she returned there around Christmas 1816; from then until her death in 1845 her concern for the cause of prisoners, and female prisoners in particular, did not slacken. In Newgate she went among the women prisoners, and spoke to them of the Gospel; she then helped them to organize schooling for their children and instruction for themselves. Together with a number of Quaker women friends, with whom she formed an Association for the Improvement of Women Prisoners in Newgate, she became a regular visitor to the prison, interesting herself in every aspect – social, moral and sanitary – of conditions of life for the female prisoners. They applied successful pressure on the authorities to appoint a female officer – a Matron – over the prisoners, and supplied them with profitable sewing work. They also worked to extend similar facilities to female convicts embarking for transportation to Australia; they eventually succeeded in obtaining the appointment of a Matron for the voyage, the provision of some instruction and occupation, and in altering existing regulations so that children under the age of seven could accompany their mothers.[2]

Contemporary literature suggests that this was the first formal association of women formed for this particular philanthropic end, though there may have been other individuals or small groups taking up similar work at the same time.[3] In 1821, when Elizabeth Fry founded the British Society, it united the local associations which had sprung up since 1817, and provided the impetus to the formation of many more: 15 British and 4 overseas associations were formed between 1821 and 1822, and by 1827 there were 34 associations in Britain and Ireland.[4] This was a movement which united women of all Protestant denominations.[5] In addition to visiting women confined in prison or awaiting transportation, these societies also concerned themselves with finding work for discharged female prisoners, or restoring them to their former homes, whether with relatives or friends.[6] In 1839 the British Society established a patronage committee to formalize this side of its work, and in 1849 The Elizabeth Fry Refuge was founded in memory of Elizabeth, who had died in 1845;[7] this provided a home for the friendless former prisoner while she searched for employment, and sometimes transferred her to another institution if a more thorough programme of personal rehabilitation under close supervision seemed called for.[8]

The competence and determination which Elizabeth Fry brought to her pastoral and administrative endeavours derived from many sources. She had been recorded as a Quaker minister in 1811, and her marriage in 1800, into a leading banking family in that community, had already placed her at the national centre of its affairs. As a young woman she had organized a school for the children of the villages attached to and surrounding her father's estate, and when mistress of her own she accepted a wide range of social responsibilities: not only supplying tenants and villagers with soup and flannel in hard winters, drugs in sickness and linen in confinements, but also, after taking instruction from the family physician Robert Willan, vaccinating the children of her parish on a regular basis.[9] In addition to these activities, which were not unusual among women of her social position,[10] Elizabeth Fry was also party to more masculine debates on social issues: I have mentioned the influence of Stephen Grellet in prompting her first prison visit, but equally important in sustaining her interest were her brother John Joseph Gurney, and her brothers-in-law Samuel Hoare and Sir Thomas Fowell Buxton, who were active in the Society for the Improvement of Prison Discipline.[11]

The core of her concern with prisons and prisoners is best stated in her own words:

> If any one wants a confirmation of the truth of Christianity, let him go and read the scriptures in prisons to poor sinners; you there see, how the gospel is exactly adapted to the fallen condition of man. It has strongly confirmed my faith, and I feel it to be, the bounden duty of the Government and the country, that those truths should be administered in the manner most likely to conduce to the real reformation of the prisoner; you then go to the root of the matter; – for though severe punishment may in a measure deter them and others from crime, it does not amend the character and change the heart.[12]

The quotation is from her evidence to the Select Committee of the House of Lords in 1835; but at the very outset of her prison career, she and John Joseph Gurney had made it clear that spiritual improvement was the supreme goal to which all merely material reforms were subordinate. In Gurney's report on the prisons which he and his sister had visited in the north and Scotland, published in 1819, we find this allusion to their great predecessor:

> Howard, indeed, drew much of the public attention to our prisons, which before his time were generally the sinks of extreme misery and terrible disease. But his efforts, and the efforts, which he excited in others, were directed more to the alleviation of distress than to the diminution of crime; more to the maintenance of the prisoner's health than to the reformation of his morals ... a judicious system of kind superintendence, of careful religious instruction, and of constant employment, was then but little contemplated. It is not, therefore, a subject of astonishment, that so many of our prisons are inadequate, in their present state, to the great purposes of reform.[13]

The central tenets of all Elizabeth Fry's reforming initiatives were rigorous and consistent. The individual was born in a state of sin, from which he or she could obtain salvation through recognizing the redemptive power of Christ. This was the meaning of reformation. For salvation and reformation to be valid, the individual had to make his or her own effort to open the heart and make the leap to God. Men and women were not machines to be remodelled, or animals to be trained. The orderly behaviour of the individual in society, though desirable, was only one manifestation of the process of reformation; the spread of Christianity, rather than the mere creation of an orderly society, was the ultimate goal. It is most important to remember that Elizabeth's definition of man as inherently sinful and tending to corruption extended to governments, Home Secretaries, Inspectors, Governors and visitors of prisons, as well as to their criminal inmates.

The watchwords of the movement which Elizabeth Fry founded and to which she gave direction and cohesion were: classification, instruction, employment, and above all, the superintendence of women by women. By the latter she meant not only that female prisoners should be guarded only by female warders, but that the warders themselves should be in some measure overseen by lady visitors. These principles of action were all directed towards the negative end of minimizing the corrupting influences of bad company and idleness, and the positive end of bringing the influence of religion, basic education and regular occupation to bear, often for the first time, on a literally captive audience.

Despite the somewhat condescending remarks about Howard just quoted, Elizabeth Fry's movement certainly did not neglect the material distress of prisoners. Elizabeth's evidence to the 1818 Commons Committee on the Prisons of the Metropolis included the assertion that the ordinary food allowance at Newgate was insufficient 'to keep any person in health' and that over a ten-month period four women and four children had died who had had only prison rations.[14] In 1827 she pointed out the dangers to prisoners of disease and cold: lack of fuel as well as lack of food was a scandal, and prisoners had been discharged 'acquitted of crime, and yet, crippled for life'.[15] In the same year the Society advised that a would-be lady visitor's first step should be to find the number of female prisoners, and the manner in which they were 'clothed, fed, attended in sickness, employed, and instructed'.[16] It was particularly important to ensure 'early medical care in cases of sickness'.[17] An undated 'Gaol Visiting Guide' which would appear to have been produced around the time of the *Observations* was specific on a number of points relating to health and sanitation: visitors were to 'See the Bread weighed occasionally', to 'examine State of Labour and Health: cause the Apothecary to attend in person generally' and to enquire: 'If Water enough? see Water Index; if in the Courts? when changed? Necessaries are cleansed? White lime used occasionally'.[18]

Nevertheless, as far as I can discover, the literature of the British Society and the visiting movement in general has very little to say specifically about the health of prisoners in general, or female prisoners in particular. I have come across surprisingly little reference to such obvious topics as childbirth in prison, or the needs of small children confined with their mothers; nor have I come across any statement on the question as to whether women should operate the treadwheel; a controversy which was almost exactly contemporary with the beginning of Elizabeth Fry's creation of a national women's organization.[19] Should we simply assume that Elizabeth's spiritual priorities diminished her interest in prisoners' physical welfare? Although this is a plausible assumption, it is worth examining a few small hints and clues in the early history of the British Society which offer a slightly different explanation.

In the sketch of their origins and progress which the ladies of the British Society published in 1827, after six years of work, Elizabeth Fry and her colleagues wrote that the Newgate ladies' 'proposals were objected to by all who dread any novelty, and were not warmly supported even by those who had made the amelioration of the condition of our species a leading object of attention'.[20] In 1828 Elizabeth was confiding to her diary her 'disappointment, from not succeeding in more generally obtaining permission for ladies to visit prisons'; and she even went so far as to say that 'of late there has been so much felt and said about our doing too much in these things with the prisoners, and going out of our province, that it makes me fearful, and consider, that as far as the Spirit is rightly subject to the prophets, so far, at this critical time, we ought to curtail in these things'.[21]

What she was describing was not, as might be thought from conventional accounts, a backlash – a sudden reversal of favour after nearly a decade of approbation. The female mission to female prisoners had in fact encountered obstacles at every stage. The comprehensive nature of the resistance is well summarized in the remarks of the outgoing Sheriff of London in 1821, expressing tolerance of visiting ladies 'so long as the Ladies Com.ee abstains from becoming parties to punishments – so long as they do nothing to censure existing laws – & confine their endeavors to the providing decent apparel – & the culture of industry and virtue'.[22]

This relegation of the ladies' work to one of clearing up existing messes and helping to maintain decency and order thereafter struck at the heart of the reforming mission. The commitment to classification did, indeed, amount to an ambitious critique of existing laws and methods of administration. Elizabeth Fry's view that a first offender should not be exposed to the vicious or hardened criminal led her to demand that prisoners should be accommodated and treated, not according to the technical offence for which they had been sentenced, but with reference to their past character. This in turn led her to question not only architectural and administrative arrangements, but the criteria of sentencing. She and her colleagues were censured for using their influence to obtain pardons and mitigations of sentences;[23] and in her *Observations* of 1827 Elizabeth, on the basis of harsh experience, warned her potential followers against attempting to obtain commutation of death penalties.[24]

It might be thought that in matters of health the ladies were on much safer ground, where they need not fear burning their fingers. But a critique in this area could also come under the heading of 'censuring existing laws'. In her *Observations*, Elizabeth recommended the visitor to use her influence to see that prison diet was adequate to maintain health and exertion, but somewhat contradictorily added that matters of diet 'are not, and ought not to be, under the control of any visiting committee of ladies'; but she insisted that the visitor should continue to exercise a good influence in assessing the capacity of prison diet to maintain health and sustain exertion.[25] Diet, as we know, was not an unproblematic aspect of prison routine, but was an essential element in the process of discipline. The calculations employed in devising a prisoner's regime involved not only financial cost and prevention of illness and debility, but also the nature of the offence, the length of the sentence, and the stage of the sentence being served.[26] For lady visitors to intervene here was certainly to depart from the domestic and aesthetic preoccupations ascribed to them and to challenge the legislative and penal functions of the state.

There is some evidence that Elizabeth Fry was warned off in another area of prison discipline which carried strong implications for women's health. The introduction of the treadwheel for female as well as male prisoners rapidly generated considerable controversy. The report that nursing mothers were put on the wheel at Guildford provoked something of an outcry at the end of 1823, and prompted the Home Office to ask all Visiting Magistrates whether this method of discipline had occasioned 'any bodily Mischief or Inconvenience'.[27] In 1824, while all of them were replying that no ill effects had been observed, William Humby, a Middlesex magistrate and medical man, was outraged to discover that a woman at Coldbath Fields House of Correction had miscarried after working on the wheel. He proposed that every female prisoner on admission should be questioned by the Matron in such a way as to prevent the possibility of pregnant women, or women who had had a very large number of confinements, being exposed to this kind of physical strain.[28]

One might have thought that this was exactly the type of administrative measure that Elizabeth Fry herself might have proposed; however, we have only two meagre pieces of evidence of her interest in this matter. The first is the record that she was, with five other ladies, given permission by the Middlesex magistrates to visit the House of Correction at Coldbath Fields between July 1825 and April 1826. At the end of that period, the Matron reported that 'on two occasions they asked and received permission to take the women from the Wheel, but this has not occurred since the first two visits'.[29] The second is a rather trenchant paragraph published a year later in a report on Irish prisons written jointly with her brother John Joseph Gurney:

> We are glad to find from the Inspectors General, that those of the other sex are never subjected to this mode of discipline. It is much better that female prisoners should be occupied under the care of ladies who visit them, with employments of a feminine and domestic nature.[30]

In 1836, the lady visitors received their strongest, most public and most official rebuke. In their report as Inspectors of Prisons for the Home District, Rev. Whitworth Russell and William Crawford strongly condemned the visitors at Newgate for acting without proper authority in matters of discipline and administration and concluded that more qualified officers should be appointed to carry out the functions which the ladies had no right to exercise.[31] By this date, legislation had consolidated several of the reforms proposed by Elizabeth, the British Society, and the SIPD, and a larger establishment of prison staff of both sexes had begun to be appointed. Elizabeth Fry's daughters, in their memoir of their mother, state that after 1836 'Her active exertions in behalf of the prisoners of the United Kingdom generally, were drawing to a close.'[32] This, as we shall see, was not true. But it was true that the British Society was undertaking more extensive work with the prisoner awaiting, or just receiving, her discharge, and that there was more official encouragement forthcoming for this than for the mission to her confined sister.

Through its Patronage Committee, through the Westminster Asylum (later renamed the Royal Female Philanthropic Society), and after Elizabeth Fry's death through the Elizabeth Fry Refuge, members of the British Society saw many women who, on release from prison, were now too ill to be rehabilitated by respectable employment. For some the ladies were able to find hospital beds; others could only be sent to the workhouse.[33] Their health before and after discharge seems to have been of relatively little interest to their benefactresses, and it is hard not to consider this an abdication from the British Society and Elizabeth Fry's earlier and larger goals. Moral rehabilitation seems to have been given priority over physical restoration, with little thought applied to the relationship between the two. One of the earliest cases in the Refuge, a Helen Grant who had served two months in Newgate for concealing the birth of a child, was observed to be 'very nervous' and in 'shaken health' while there; after only a week she was found a post in service, from which she was dismissed a month later for 'total refusal to obey or perform the duties assigned her'. Two weeks later she was in Guy's Hospital, suffering from pleurisy. Her history does not seem to have prompted any soul-searching or discussion of physiological cause and behavioural effect.[34]

The management of the Refuge itself appears to have endorsed prevailing conditions in the prisons which the women had left. The dietary proposed for the newly released inmates by Elizabeth Fry's daughter Katharine was rejected as 'if anything rather too liberal', and the ladies of the House Committee 'were requested to procure dietaries from prisons and Union Houses'.[35] The erection of partitions between beds in order to ensure 'a more strict system of classification in the sleeping rooms' reduced ventilation so drastically that the medical officers appointed by the (male) General Committee insisted on their removal.[36] In the circumstances, it was hardly to be expected that the British Society would pass comment on, let alone criticize the prison facilities which delivered women to the Refuge in a poor state of health. Worse, the deaths of many of these women were exploited, most egregiously by Matilda Wrench in a publication of 1852, to illustrate the gloriously happy endings to which the pastoral ministrations of the ladies had conduced.[37] Even if they had felt a more lively concern over health issues, the ladies of the British Society could not have afforded to antagonize the authorities; the visitors had no official standing in the prisons, and any controversy would have jeopardized their activities. At the same time, the Society, in appealing for public subscriptions, was under some pressure to prove that it could achieve reformatory results; and it was at least true that the dead could go out and sin no more.

The last decade or so of Elizabeth Fry's life was one of immense activity in a great variety of philanthropic fields, including nursing reform and the district visiting movement.[38] Her prison concerns were most conspicuously displayed in visits to the Continent. However, she continued to press for reform at home, and began to concentrate her efforts more and more on one particular issue, that of solitary confinement. In her early work at Newgate, and her joint writings with John Joseph Gurney, she had given some sanction to this form of punishment. By 1834 her opposition was becoming increasingly pronounced.[39] It was rooted in some of her deepest and earliest personal experiences, confirmed and shaped by her religious convictions.

It is, indeed, impossible to read the meditations in Elizabeth's diary without recalling Gerard Manley Hopkins' lines in his *No Worst, There is None*: 'O, the mind, mind has mountains; ... Hold them cheap/ May who ne'er hung there'. Two entries may be quoted out of hundreds. Shortly before her marriage, in August 1800, she wrote: 'It is a blessing indeed to feel thus healthy in mind and body; for I think we are subject to mental diseases that are not in our power, any more than bodily ones, and that require our patience; although it is our duty in both mental and bodily maladies to overcome them.' And in May 1803, after the birth of her second child: 'I have gone through much since, in various ways, from real bodily weakness, and also the trials of a nervous imagination: no one knows but those who have felt them, how hard they are to bear, for they lead the mind to look for trouble, and it requires much exertion not to be led away by them; nothing I believe allays them so much as the quieting influence of religion.'[40]

Throughout the 1830s and 1840s her empirical observations of the effects of solitary confinement confirmed her in these views of the relationship between body, mind and soul. As she wrote in 1838 to the Aberdeen authorities: 'The opinion I had previously formed, as to the peculiar care required in applying this system, was confirmed by learning, on visiting your prison, that no less than two of the prisoners, now in confinement, had attempted self-destruction.' In April 1841 she noted in her diary of a visit to a transport ship 'several of the poor women having become delirious from the excitement of the change from separate confinement to the bustle of the ship. This must lead me to make further and stronger efforts for an entire change of the system adopted with them.'[41]

Although she was willing to concede that a prisoner returning on a second charge should then be confined separately, having instruction and employment, and a certain number of visits daily,[42] her primary concern was that the mental health of the prisoner should be nurtured as carefully as his or her physical health; and that mental health was as conducive to reformation as its absence was productive of criminality. In 1841 she wrote urgently to Joshua Jebb in an attempt to persuade him to alter the design of the cells planned for Pentonville:

> I am certain that separate confinement produces an unhealthy state, both of mind and body, and that, therefore, everything should be done to counteract this influence, which, I am sure, is baneful in its moral tendency; for I am satisfied that a sinful course of life increases the tendency to mental derangement, as well as bodily disease; ... the mind in an enervated state is more liable to yield to temptation, than when in a lively powerful state; and I consider light, air, and the power of seeing something beyond the mere monotonous walls of a cell, highly important. I am aware that air is properly admitted, also light, still I do think they ought to see the sky, the changes in which make it a most pleasant object for those closely confined. ... I do not believe that a despairing or stupefied state is suitable for leading poor sinners to a Saviour's feet for pardon and salvation.[43]

Later that year, all too conscious of the fact that the seed was falling on stony ground, she used the occasion of a Mansion House dinner to take her complaints to the top, expressing to Prince Albert 'my fear that our punishments were becoming too severe – my wish that the Queen should be informed of some particulars respecting separate confinement' and begged Sir Robert Peel to see the New Prison, and 'to have the dark cells a little altered'.[44]

That she failed utterly to make an impact on official policy on solitary confinement is a clear sign that Elizabeth Fry's mission had fallen out of the main current of prison reform, and that a secular, behavioural strategy and a policy of deterrence for habitual offenders now took precedence over her own agenda of individual salvation and the Christianizing, or re-Christianizing, of society. But this defeat was not simply an outcome of the conflict between religious and secular ideals of reformation. It is most unlikely that, if Elizabeth Fry had couched her arguments on the relationship between mental health and criminality in purely secular terms, her views on solitary confinement would have received more respectful attention. For she was moved to protest, not just by her own profound psychological insights, but by a radical and fundamental critique of the state in its penal capacity. Religious in its origin, it could not be contained within a conventional framework of rendering unto Caesar.

In an address to a Scottish audience in 1838, reported by her daughters, she gave an uncompromising exposition of her views:

> She shrank from the abuses to which the solitary system is liable. How soon might the cell become an oubliette; how short the transition from kind and constant attention, to cruelty and neglect; how entirely the comfort, nay the existence of a prisoner, must depend upon his keeper's will; and what was human nature, to be trusted with such responsibility? with an active magistracy, a zealous clergyman, and careful medical attendant, all might be well; but who could ensure the continuance of the advantages? and were the activity and benevolence of the present day to pass away, why might not the slumber of indifference again cover the land? Nor was this her only fear – 'They may be building, though they little think it, dungeons for their children and their children's children, if times of religious persecution or political disturbance should return.' Cell within cell, as in some prisons, in others the light and air of heaven admitted through a crooked funnel, but the glorious sun shut from their eyes; with no sound to reach them; and, – but a keeper withdrawn, or a wire broken, – no sound to be heard from them, however deep the need of assistance.[45]

And her letter to Jebb of 1841 echoed this theme:

> however lenient those who now govern, we can little calculate upon the change the future may produce, ... my experience most strongly proves, that there are few men who are themselves sufficiently governed and regulated by Christian principle, to be fit to have such power entrusted in their hands; and further, I observe, that officers in prisons have generally so much to try and to provoke them, that they themselves are apt to become hardened to the more tender feelings of humanity; they necessarily, also, see so much through the eyes of those under them, turnkeys and inferior officers (too many of whom are little removed, either in education or morals, from the prisoners themselves,) that their judgements are not always just.[46]

How, it might be asked, could such a voice possibly become the voice of authority? How could it be identified with the mainstream of nineteenth-century reform, which depended so confidently on the premise that a suitable body of legislation, proper administrative machinery, the right architecture, and the oversight of a Chaplain of the Church of England would be sufficient to prosper most institutions within the body politic? Perhaps it should not surprise us to read, in Howard Association pamphlets and elsewhere, that by the early 1870s both male and female prison visitors felt that there was an official tendency to discourage their activities, or at the very least not to encourage them.[47] This tendency was accentuated after the nationalization of the prison service in 1877, when many women who had been visiting their local prisons for years found vague objections being raised by Governors, and their activities put on hold.[48] Susanna Meredith, who had begun visiting work at Millbank under the auspices of the British Society in 1858 and who undertook independent work at Brixton around 1865, found her activities, never free of official resistance, abruptly curtailed in 1877.[49] She recalled nearly two decades later that on being refused permission to speak to women prisoners in the absence of the matron: 'I said, "Then I will not go any more".'[50]

Voluntary visiting in prisons, and women's philanthropic work for prisoners, did not die out in 1877, although the scope of visitors' work, and their freedom to comment on policy, were severely restricted. Non-denominational bodies such as the Discharged Prisoners' Aid Society and the Howard Association, as well as denominational ones (Mrs Meredith was associated with the deaconess movement), all of which recruited much voluntary womanpower, played a large role in continuing and developing work in this field. The advantages and disadvantages of lady visitors were rediscovered and rehearsed at many points in the second half of the century, and a new national Lady Visitors' Association was formed with official sanction under the presidency of the Duchess of Bedford in 1901. It was later renamed the National Association of Visitors to Women Prisoners; at the end of the Second World War it fused with its male opposite number to form the National Association of Prison Visitors.[51]

When Susanna Meredith recalled for the Parliamentary Commission of 1894 the circumstances in which she withdrew from prison visiting in 1877, she added a most revealing insight into the privileged *modus operandi* of some lady volunteers: before the latter date she had reported on her activities and observations directly to Sir George Grey, the Home Secretary.[52] It cannot be wondered at that this channel of communication should have fallen victim to the increased formalization and professionalization of the prison service. That it should ever have existed at all is a reminder of the slowness of these developments within mny branches of the public services in Victorian Britain; obvious comparisons may be made with the privileged lines of communication between Sidney Herbert at the War Office and the lady volunteer Florence Nightingale at Scutari 1854–6, and between the first (unsalaried) lady superintendent of army nurses and the Secretary of State for War 1861–8.[53]

Without the evidence of Elizabeth Fry's protests, it would be easy enough to dismiss the narrative of the limitation and marginalization of women's visiting work in prisons simply as that of the unequal contest between voluntarism and amateurism on the one hand, and bureaucratization and professionalization on the other. But, as we have seen, deeper values than organizational ones were in collision. Elizabeth Fry's dissidence was not enunciated by her female successors in terms of an anti-state critique; but it was perpetuated by deeds as well as words which upheld a view of the purposes of imprisonment and the moral potential of prisoners radically different from that which was becoming the official norm.

In 1862 Catherine Frazer, who as a young woman had accompanied Elizabeth Fry on her visits, had this to say to the National Association for the Promotion of Social Science about the female inmates of Millbank:

> Great allowance should be made for persons who have lost self-respect and yet retain that love of approbation which is so natural to the human mind. They have no happy thoughts, no right principles of action within, and they look abroad for somebody who will place them on better terms with themselves; this is the secret of many outbreaks among prisoners. The mind preys upon itself till reflection becomes intolerable. They sometimes appear to have a kind of savage joy in incurring punishment, because they know they will thus obtain notice, and give trouble to their officers and gratify some of their chosen companions.... Does not this show the advantage of holding as far as possible individual communication with these poor girls, and thus striving to induce them to seek the approval of those who earnestly desire to promote their best interests and to raise them from the depths of degradation into which they are plunging themselves?

She insisted that real incorrigibility was rare, and was to be taken as evidence of feebleness of mind.[54]

While Catherine Frazer was expressing these views to the National

Association, those in authority were making very different statements in their evidence on women deemed 'out of control' to the Royal Commission on Penal Servitude. William Augustus Guy, the Medical Superintendent at Millbank, stated: 'I think if it were possible to inflict upon them some short bodily pain, it would be much more merciful', and Captain D. O'Brien, a Director of Convict Prisons, declared that 'they become so utterly depraved, and so detestable in every way that really I can hardly speak of them with common equanimity'.[55] This was the language of ankle straps and padded cells; it offered little scope for the kind of interaction Frazer described:

> It is often better to lead them to relate some passages of their early life by way of getting at their real state of mind, than to question them as to their later experience. It lately happened that one of the ladies who was visiting a prisoner at Millbank, inquired from whence she had come, and what her employment had been, before she had got into prison. She said she had worked in the Staffordshire potteries and could earn ten or twelve shillings per week. She then began to describe the process of turning the clay by means of a wheel into a circular form. Some very simple questions seemed suddenly to bring back to her recollection her days of comparative innocence, and she burst into tears. She was considered a hardened prisoner, and at that time was in the penal class, but there was truth and feeling in those tears, such as could not perhaps have been elicited by more direct means. It is the great aim of the visitors to these poor outcasts to bring some element of truth into their hearts and consciences. The more they can be individualized the better ...[56]

It was an old quarrel. When the British Society ladies had first received permission to visit Millbank in 1836, the Superintending Committee of the penitentiary attached a set of conditions to the privilege, of which the sixth ran 'that while the Ladies manifest the kindness and gentleness dictated by their Christian principles and by their sex, they will always bear in mind, that the persons visited are Prisoners sentenced by the Law to a state of punishment, and that it is incumbent upon those who converse with them to repress every thing approaching to undue familiarity'. Elizabeth Fry and her associates immediately 'proposed that an explanation of the 6th resolution be requested of the Gentlemen's Committee'.[57] Twenty-six years later, as Catherine Frazer's account shows, the British Society was still doggedly pressing its case against an increasingly resistant officialdom.

However discreet and tactful Elizabeth Fry's successors and disciples in the prison visiting movement might be, however fulsome in their acknowledgement of the kindness of magistrates, inspectors, governors and officers of prisons, the very fact of visiting – especially throughout the duration of a sentence, rather than just before discharge – was a continual reminder that inmates were individuals, with experiences and identities which extended beyond the set of definitions inspired by organizational and disciplinary imperatives. The existence of the visitors was an irritant and a challenge to the system as it developed in the latter part of the nineteenth century. Perhaps the British Society's most abiding legacy to the discussion of the health of prisoners was its dual contention that prisoners of disturbed mind required better treatment, and that prison conditions were in themselves a causal or aggravating factor in mental disturbance.

In 1827, Elizabeth Fry introduced her *Observations on the Visiting, Superintendence and Government of Female Prisons* by saying that the previous ten years had demonstrated the success of female philanthropic work in prisons; and she called for it to be extended to hospitals, lunatic asylums and workhouses. There were only 'comparatively solitary instances in which women, in our own country, have been in the habit of regularly visiting the public abodes of poverty or disease'.[58] One of her British Society successors, Matilda Wrench, repeated this call in 1852: 'It is much to be desired that the system which has done so much for the prisoners might be extended to the sick and the poor in our workhouses and hospitals. ... Many are dissatisfied with a life of aimless ease. HERE IS WORK TO BE DONE!'[59]

The relative success of Elizabeth Fry and her associates in gaining entry to a secular public institution undoubtedly gave enormous encouragement to other women to enter other public institutions; it might even be argued that the frustration of many of the prison visitors' ambitions provided the impetus for women to assault more accessible citadels:[60] to take into workhouses the principle that gentlewomen should care for the wretched of their own sex, and that the poor, especially the female poor, should be classified and segregated to avoid the moral contamination of the merely wretched by the plainly vicious. The most important application of that principle, and the one which had the greatest bearing on the development of national medical services, was that whereby accommodation was provided for the sick, infirm or deranged poor separately from that provided for other recipients of relief, and, ultimately, without the stigma of pauperization. In hospitals, the principle that working women should be supervised by voluntary or salaried ladies was already operative within the Anglican sisterhood movement by the date of Matilda Wrench's appeal, and was to be secularized a decade later with the establishment of the Nightingale Training School.

Although Elizabeth Fry was not able to make the contribution that she herself wished to either the physical or mental health of prisoners, she undoubtedly inspired, directly and indirectly, the work of spiritual god-daughters such as Louisa Twining and Florence Nightingale which was to redefine standards of care for the sick poor at large.

Notes

1. The most recent biography is June Rose's *Elizabeth Fry* (London, 1980); Janet Whitney's *Elizabeth Fry, Quaker Heroine* (London, 1937) remains a valuable study. Both works are referenced, but without footnotes.
2. *Memoir of the life of Elizabeth Fry*, ed. Katharine Fry and Rachel E. Cresswell (London, 1847), 2 v., (henceforward *Memoir*) is the most detailed printed source on all Elizabeth Fry's work for prisoners; see also Lucia Zedner, *Women, Crime and Custody in Victorian England* (Oxford, 1991).
3. Sarah Martin, a dressmaker of Yarmouth, whose mission to prisons was almost exactly contemporaneous with that of Elizabeth Fry, and who worked as an individual, though in contact with the British Society, is probably the best known of these: see George Mogridge, *Sarah Martin the Prison-Visitor* (London: Religious Tract Society, 1872).
4. *Sketch of the Origin and Results of Ladies Prison Associations* (London, 1827), 19–20, 43, 49.
5. The minutes of the British Society reveal incidents of friction between Protestant and Roman Catholic lady visitors in Ireland in 1828, and of disruption of Protestant prayer meetings by Catholic women prisoners in Millbank and Brixton convict prisons in 1863: Hackney Archive (henceforward HA) D/S 58 3/1, British Society Minutes 30.6.28, D/S 58 3/2, Minutes 19.10.63.
6. C. Frazer, 'The British Ladies Society for Female Prisoners', *Transactions of the National Association for the Promotion of Social Science*, 1862, 496; see also Greater London Record Office (henceforward GLRO) M/F OC/21, Middlesex Sessions Records, f. 489, report of Chaplain, 30.3.1826.
7. Rather surprisingly, the initiative to found the refuge was taken in February 1846, not by the British Society, but by a group of male friends and associates including Edward Buxton, Lord Ashley and the Chevalier de Bunsen; it was some months before they accepted the ladies of the British Society as equal partners in the venture. HA D/S 58 1/1, Elizabeth Fry Refuge General Committee Minutes, 30.4.46.
8. Matilda Wrench, *Visits to Female Prisons at Home and Abroad* (London, 1852), 116.
9. *Memoir* I, 172.
10. On the range of such activities, see F.K. Prochaska, *Women and*

Philanthropy in 19th Century England (Oxford, 1980).

11. On the relationship between the ideas of Elizabeth Fry and those of the SIPD, see R.A. Cooper, 'Jeremy Bentham, Elizabeth Fry and Prison Reform', *Journal of the History of Ideas*, 42, 1981, 675–90.
12. *Memoir* II, 208–9.
13. J.J. Gurney, *Notes on a visit made to some of the Prisons in Scotland and the North of England, in company with Elizabeth Fry* (London, 1819), 98–9.
14. *Report from the Committee on the Prisons of the Metropolis, PP* 1818 VIII, 333.
15. E. Fry, *Observations on the Visiting, Superintendence and Government of Female Prisons* (London, 1827), 62.
16. *Sketch*, 49.
17. E. Fry, *Observations*, 55.
18. Bodleian Library, John Johnson Collection, *Prisons*, Box 3.
19. Webb, Sidney, and Webb, Beatrice, *English Prisons under Local Government* (1922), 97–8.
20. *Sketch*, 5–6.
21. *Memoir* I, 61–2.
22. British Library (henceforward BL) Eg. MS. 3673 A, ff. 180v–181.
23. *Report of Inspectors of Prisons of Great Britain for the Home District, PP* 1836 XXXV, 22.
24. E. Fry, *Observations*, 24.
25. *Ibid.*, 56.
26. For an extended treatment of this topic, see the contribution to this volume by Anne Hardy.
27. Public Record Office (henceforward PRO) HO 20/2, (no foliation).
28. PRO HO 20/2, letters and notebook of Humby.
29. GLRO, M/F OC/21, Middlesex Sessions Records, f. 490, report for 13.4.26.
30. *Report addressed to the Marquess Wellesley, Lord Lieutenant of Ireland, by Elizabeth Fry and John Joseph Gurney, respecting their late Visit to that Country* (London, 1827), 14.
31. *Report of Inspectors of Prisons of Great Britain for the Home District, PP* 1836 XXXV, 17, 21–2.
32. *Memoir* II, 230.
33. Wrench, *op. cit.*, 23, 74, 126; Frazer, *op. cit.*, 500.
34. HA D/S 58 1/14, Elizabeth Fry Refuge, Case Book c.1849–54, f. 4.
35. HA D/S 58 1/2, Elizabeth Fry Refuge, House Committee Minutes 16.11.49, 3.1.50.
36. HA D/S 58 1/2, Elizabeth Fry Refuge, House Committee Minutes 25.6.50; HA D/S 58 1/1, Elizabeth Fry Refuge, General Committee Minutes, 14.12.52.
37. Wrench, *op.cit.*, 45 *et seq.*
38. *Memoir* II, *passim*; C.C. Southey (ed.), *The Life and*

Correspondence of the Late Robert Southey (London, 1850), vol. VI, 66–9; Rev. J. Aspinall, *A Sermon preached at St. Michael's Church, Liverpool, ... upon the subject of the Provident District Society* (Liverpool, 1830), 6; *Hints on District Visiting Societies* (London: Longmans, 1836), 50–6; A. Summers, 'The costs and benefits of caring: nursing charities *c.*1830–*c.*1860' in Jonathan Barry and Colin Jones (eds), *Medicine and Charity before the Welfare State* (London: Routledge, 1991).

39. *Memoir* II, 198.
40. *Memoir* I, 92, 114–15.
41. *Memoir* II, 282, 387.
42. *Memoir* II, 309–10, 313.
43. *Memoir* II, 396.
44. *Memoir* II, 423.
45. *Memoir* II, 287.
46. *Memoir* II, 395–6.
47. William Tallack, *The Cellular (But.NOT rigidly solitary) System of Imprisonment* (London: Howard Association, 1872); Amelia Lewis, 'Fulham Prison for Females', *Woman*, 10.2.72, 62–3. For a summary account of the progressive limitations placed on women's visiting, see Prochaska, *op.cit.*, 169–73.
48. PRO HO 45/956S/75257, correspondence of July and August 1880.
49. HA D/S 58 3/2, British Society Minutes 22.3.58, 16.12.67.
50. *Report of the Departmental Committee on Prisons, PP* 1895 LVI, 246. For an extended account of her religious and philanthropic career, see M.A. Lloyd, *Susanna Meredith* (London, 1903).
51. Sheila R. Lochhead, *Outside-in: A Study of Prison Visiting* (York: William Sessions, 1993).
52. HA D/S 58 3/2, British Society Minutes 16.12.67; *Report of the Departmental Committee on Prisons, PP* 1895 LVI, 246.
53. A. Summers, *Angels and Citizens; British Women as Military Nurses 1854–1914* (Routledge, 1988), ch. 3. The privileged relationship with the Secretary of State had largely disappeared by 1878; *ibid.*, 98–9.
54. Frazer, *op.cit.*, 497–8.
55. Royal Commission on Penal Servitude, *PP* 1863 XXI, 532, 458.
56. Frazer, *op.cit.*, 499.
57. HA D/S 58 3/1, British Society Minutes 19.12.36.
58. E. Fry, *Observations*, 5.
59. Wrench, *op.cit.*, 98.
60. See also Prochaska, *op.cit.*, 173.

Commentary

Summers (In response to a question) I think Elizabeth Fry suffered from depression. She had eleven confinements and was wretchedly ill after every one of them. But I think that she was volatile, quite fragile: that is why she kept such a voluminous diary. The problem with diaries is that you are longing to hear her say what she did in Newgate, but she uses her diary to discuss the problems of the day and the problems of her soul. There is no record in the diary of her being rebuked over the treadwheel incident because that is the time when her husband is approaching bankruptcy and her standing in the community is at stake. You are often very frustrated; on the other hand the diaries are a very great source for understanding her empathy with other beings under pressure.

6

The Prison Medical Service and the Deviant 1895 – 1948

Joe Sim

In this chapter I want to provide a critical dissection and analysis of prison health care between 1895, the year when the Gladstone Committee reported and 1948, the year when the Criminal Justice Act was passed. This was also the year when the National Health Service (NHS) was established in the United Kingdom. These dates and events have not been picked at random. As I shall indicate, both the Gladstone Report and the Criminal Justice Act had profound implications for the Prison Medical Service (PMS) and the confined. The development of the NHS was also important in that prison medical care was excluded from the clauses which established free universal health care for all UK subjects irrespective of their social status. Despite the establishment of the NHS the delivery of health care for the confined remained under the managerial control of the Home Office rather than being placed with the newly established network of nationalized health boards.

Before considering the sociology of prison medicine between these two dates it is also important to recognize that by 1895 the PMS already had over 100 years of history, experience and controversy behind it. This controversy as I have argued elsewhere was focused around two interrelated areas (Sim 1990). First, there was the relationship between prison doctors and the broader regulatory concerns of penal institutions. This relationship very often involved the subsumption of medical care to disciplinary penality which in turn was underpinned by the doctrine of 'less eligibility'. According to many social commentators, including doctors, prisoners could not receive medical care that was equivalent to or better than the care that those outside the walls of the penitentiary received. Second, there was the issue of the involvement of doctors in the management of individual prisoners and prison regimes in general. Indeed in the fifteen years before Gladstone reported, as Alison Liebling and Tony Ward illustrate in Chapter 7, there were a series of controversial deaths in custody which highlighted the role of medical personnel in the dietary management of prisoners and the articulation of the principles of 'less eligibility' by a number of prison doctors dressed in the language of scientific study and debate. Similarly while this paper stops in 1948 the issues around health care for the confined and the role of medical personnel in the management of individuals and institutions have continued to reverberate into the 1990s. In the four decades since 1948 a range of questions have been asked by politicians, prisoners' rights organizations, media personnel, official medical bodies and prisoners themselves about the standard of prison health care, conditions in prison hospitals, the training of hospital officers, the use of psychotropic drugs as mechanisms of control, the lack of health and safety provisions behind the walls and the differential treatment of women and Afro-Caribbean prisoners (*ibid*: chs 5 and 6). It is important to bear these points in mind before focusing on the years between 1895 and 1948.

Sociological Issues and Theoretical Concerns

There are three issues I want to explore in this chapter. First, there is the general question of the physical and psychological health of prisoners in the period under consideration and the ideologies that those who worked in the PMS brought to their work. Second, there are the views of prisoners themselves and how they saw their relationship with the PMS. This issue has been dominated by the voices of the powerful and the hierarchy of credibility within which they operate. Prisoners' voices have until recently been marginalized and yet they provide a poignant and alternative account of the place of medicine in the penitentiary. Finally, there is the relationship between medical power and gender and the differential treatment accorded to the female deviant between 1895 and 1948.

In exploring these sociological issues I shall utilize a theoretical framework deriving from the work of Michel Foucault and in particular Foucault's insistence on the need to understand the development of medical and psychiatric discourses in relation to the exercise of power and its effects. Central to Foucault's project (and that of other social theorists such as Zygmunt Bauman, Jurgen Habermas and Nils Christie) is the rejection of the Enlightenment vision of rational progress and benevolent development which has dominated social scientific discourse about modern institutions in general and medicine in particular. Instead Foucault ties the genesis of modernity into the emergence, construction and consolidation of a disciplinary society in which increasing numbers of individuals and groups are subjected to its punitive gaze. Integral to the process of disciplinary power are discourses of surveillance, individualization and normalization.

It is my contention that the history of the PMS in general and its development between 1895 and 1948 in particular is best understood within this theoretical framework. Rather than the development of the PMS being understood as a series of evolutionary, benevolent reforms underpinned by the march of scientific progress, I want to argue that those who have staffed the PMS have, with honourable exceptions, been concerned with not only normalizing prisoners through the discipline of less eligibility but have also been concerned with maintaining the order of individual institutions and contributing to the policing of more general social divisions. Prison medical workers have done this through their unique access to, and surveillance of the confined. Within the prison, as Foucault called it 'that darkest region in the apparatus of justice' prisoners were broken down and fragmented into individual cellular spaces 'thus allowing their control and ordering through routines and time-tables' (Patton 1979: 121). The consolidation of prison medicine and its knowledge base reinforced this fragmentation as constant surveillance and individualized documentation became corner-stones in penality. Medical knowledge, in other words, regulated 'the exercise of penitentiary practice' (Foucault 1977: 250). This knowledge was part of a disciplinary project oriented to:

> creating a model individual, conducting his life according to the precepts of health, and creating a medicalized society in order to bring the conditions of life and conduct in line with the requirements of health. (Cousins and Hussain 1984: 151)

As I have argued elsewhere, the prison:

> became a laboratory in which the advice and expertise of the medical profession, both physicians and psychiatrists, was geared to reintegrating the confined back to normality. Domination through observation objectified the prisoner ... probing, testing, studying and examining the bod[ies] and mind[s] of the confined was intrinsic to the development of power relationships. (Sim, *op. cit.*: 9)

It is within this theoretical framework that the three issues I discussed earlier will be addressed.

Prisoners' Health and Social Discipline

As I noted above the health care of prisoners has been determined by the discourses of less eligibility since the genesis of the PMS in 1774. Over the next 120 years, prison doctors as a body of professionals despite different emphases and nuances articulated quite precise views about the nature of criminality and deviance and the interventions that were needed to stem the tide of illegality and disorder which appeared ready to break through the dyke of morality erected by respectable society and drown an increasingly supine and defenceless social body. The assertion and imposition of discipline within and without the walls of the penitentiary was central to stemming this tide. As Dr Thornton, a prison medical officer wrote in *The Lancet* in March 1895:

> It is not always remembered by writers that the inmates of a prison are largely made up of the scum of our population ready for any disturbance if the government is lax, and lax prison management is not a kindness, nor is it safe. (*The Lancet*, 30 March 1895: 839)

By this time, prison doctors, along with a range of other newly emerging professional groups were concerned with differentiating the conditions which were conducive to the genesis of criminality and disorder. In October 1895, Dr Gover, the Medical Inspector of Prisons, wrote in *The Lancet* that:

> the criminal elements in society may be largely reduced by such social reforms as the prevention of overcrowding, by attention to the details of sanitation, by judicious education and by such training as will tend to eradicate habits of idleness. (*The Lancet*, 12 October 1895: 911)

This concern with rescuing the confined from the criminal abyss reflected the broader debates about the remoralisation of the idle, the poor and the criminal and through this process reasserting the moral health of the society. (Garland 1985).

Dr Gover's paper appeared in the same year that the Gladstone Committee reported. Liberal analyses of this report have consistently articulated the view that the Committee's recommendations on treatment and training mark the beginning of the modern prison's desire to reform the prisoner. However, a critical reading of the report reveals a more complex picture. As Peter Young has noted Gladstone's proposals were 'yoked to the more mundane demands of prison discipline ... reform and discipline were collapsed to mean the same thing' (Young 1983: 97). A number of prison doctors provided their own evidence to the Committee which referred to the 'degenerate stock' from which criminals came, their moral insanity and their 'furtive eyes' (Gatrell 1980: 83). According to Martin Wiener most medical officers favoured 'some sort of medical treatment' for professional criminals 'of flexible duration, either curative or incapacitative' (Wiener 1990: 347).

For the purposes of this paper what is important about Gladstone is not only the disciplinary concerns articulated by prison doctors but also that the report extended the power of medical personnel in prisons. When the Prison Act was passed in 1898 which enacted Gladstone's proposals it was clear that the role of the prison doctor had developed considerably both in relation to supporting 'the governor in the maintenance of discipline and order' (Prison Commissioners 1898: 29) and in the areas of psychiatric examination, classification and disposal. By the turn of the century while the status of the prison doctors remained low and while there were continuous conflicts with the Home Office over pay and conditions, their role in dealing with prisoners classified as insane and mentally deficient, in writing pre-sentence reports, in publishing a range of literature and in teaching and attending conferences increased dramatically. By 1922 Dr Norwood East who was later to become Medical Inspector of Prisons was producing 700 to 800 reports a year on the mental condition of prisoners (Watson 1988: 133).

While these developments might be understood as an indication of the progress of medical and psychiatric knowledge, I want to argue that they also have to be understood within the broader disciplinary context I discussed earlier. There were a number of dimensions to this. First, the doctors were still heavily involved in the development of regulatory regimes for those prisoners classified as difficult. In December 1904, Dr Smalley the Medical Inspector of Prisons discussed the strengths and weaknesses of different strategies of control. These he termed 'chemical', 'mechanical' and 'plenty of attendants' (Sim, *op. cit.*: 66). Second, Smalley and other doctors were involved in the broader debates around social problems and social hygiene. The Royal Commission on the Care and Control of the Feeble-Minded which reported in 1908 included amongst its members Dr Horatio Donkin who was the Medical Commissioner of Prisons. As David Garland has noted the Mental Deficiency Act which followed in 1913 was concerned with the threat that the increase in the number of feeble-minded posed to society. This in turn meant:

> the extension of the role of state, which becomes the subject of wider and more penetrating forms of social regulation; promoting expertise and the accumulation of disciplinary knowledge; and the

> establishment of practices of individualisation, accompanied by rhetorics of reform. (Garland, *op. cit.*: 225)

Smalley himself had pursued a similar line arguing for the permanent detention of the feeble-minded in a 'suitable institution' (Sim, *op. cit.*: 67). Recent research has pointed to the often detrimental impact that this detention engendered particularly for feeble-minded women who were regarded as more fertile than their normal sisters. Dr Gill the first Medical Superintendent of Calderstones Asylum in Lancashire, had his professional roots in prison medicine and gave evidence to the 1934 Royal Commission into Sterilization (The Brock Report). Gill called for eugenic sterilization for the 'mentally deficient'. While these policies were not pursued in the UK, doctors like Gill supported harsh and disciplinary regimes like Calderstones for the regulation and control of the mentally deficient. As Susan O'Malley and Gillian Hall (1988) have noted the regimes had a dire impact on the lives of those detained in them. Many of these individuals were detained for decades often at the discretion of the Medical Superintendent whose professional expertise was unassailable within the institution's hierarchy.

Medicine from Below

In considering the development of prison medicine since Gladstone it is important in my view to point to how those who were interacting with the PMS – the prisoners – understood their role. Prisoners' accounts of life inside still remain a neglected and marginalized area, the construction of penal 'truth' in the Foucauldian sense having emanated from the powerful whose account of historical events has become the accepted history of penality. And yet from the late nineteenth century a series of autobiographical accounts emerged which told a very different story from the journey to medical nirvana which has dominated conventional histories. With the publication of *English Prisons Today* in 1922 these accounts were conveyed to a much wider audience. This book, written by Stephen Hobhouse and Fenner Brockway, presented a 728-page analysis of the state of English prisons between 1914 and 1919. Based on prisoners' accounts of life inside it was particularly critical of the PMS. The authors found that medical care and treatment of the sick was inadequate; prison hospitals were used for solitary confinement; there was no hospital treatment in small prisons; there was a relationship between the lack of medical care and deaths in custody; doctors had little or no training in classifying mental illness; finally doctors were involved in investigating 'shamming' and were allowed on the authority of the Visiting Committee or a Commissioner to apply a 'painful test' to the prisoners involved. They would be placed in a shower bath surrounded by iron bars, the temperature of the water plus the iron bars being designed to make the individual 'confess to the doctor that he is shamming and so escape further treatment' (Hobhouse and Brockway 1922: 261).

The research conducted by Hobhouse and Brockway was supported by the writings of a number of prisoners which appeared in the 1930s and 1940s. The autobiographies of Wilfred Macartney and Red Collar Man published in the mid-1930s described in grim detail the standard of medical care, the superficial nature of medical examinations and the involvement of doctors in a number of disciplinary duties. Macartney came into contact with nine doctors and 'with one or two exceptions they impressed the prisoner as a heartless and indolent and incompetent crew' (Macartney 1936: 103). Red Collar Man's autobiography told a similar story. He maintained that the doctors 'with few exceptions are very callous in jail'. He pointed to their involvement in disciplinary activities including flogging where the man's back was 'covered with long red weals and the skin is broken and bloody. These marks never fade right out, but remain for life' (Red Collar Man 1937: 155). Similar stories were told in the 1940s by prisoners and ex-prisoners.

The situation became so serious that the Prison Medical Reform Council (PMRC) was formed. In 1943, the Council published a pamphlet entitled *Prison Medical Service* which identified 'grave defects in the Prison Medical Service'. These defects included: assuming that every prisoner was a malingerer, providing medical treatment that was perfunctory and casual and supporting provision for dental care that was 'callously inadequate' (Prison Medical Reform Council 1943a: 3–4). In the same year the PMRC published an account of life for women in Holloway. Again the medical examination was 'so superficial it is a wonder that any disease is ever diagnosed'. Pregnant women were locked in their cells each night in solitary confinement 'right up to the time the baby [was] due' (Prison Medical Reform Council 1943b: 21–2). I shall return to the question of medicine and confined women below. For the moment it is important to note that the PMRC's work continued the tradition established by Hobhouse and Brockway and was to be followed by a range of prisoners' rights organizations over the next four decades. At the same time its work took place in the context of a changing social and political landscape which was established in the aftermath of the Second World War. For many commentators the period after 1945 marks a distinct watershed in the evolution of British society towards a more welfare-oriented system. Clearly the establishment of the NHS was a great leap forward for many in society compared with the often appalling discretionary and costly delivery of medical treatment prior to 1948. How much of a watershed this period became for prisoners and their health remains a matter of debate.

National Health and the Exclusion of the Confined

Space does not allow for a thorough examination of the developments in post-war British society. This I have done elsewhere (Sim 1989: ch. 3). It is important to note that state intervention through groups of professionals, was a central element in the social reconstructionist ideology of the period. The medical profession, overwhelmingly white and male, was a powerful and well-organized voice in the debates about crime and penal policy. Prison doctors (and eventually prison psychologists) increasingly set the parameters for debates about crime and criminality. There were a number of complex reasons for this. First, there was the medical profession's forceful ideological claim that it could root out the causes of crime. Second, there was the apparent rise in crime itself which doctors and psychologists claimed could be halted if they were given the freedom to research and experiment. Third, the nature of the social democratic consensus built on the ideologies of welfarism, interventionism and professional expertise provided the bridgehead that consolidated the expansion of medical influence within and without institutions.

Theories of criminality propagated by the medical profession and by professionals in general clustered around a number of themes: the impact of the war and the question of the physical environment, family disorganization, individual psychopathology and in the case of black people sexuality and miscegenation. What should be done taxed the collective minds of both professional medical people and intellectuals of the time.

The prison was central to this debate particularly the kind of regimes that prisoners should experience. The institution itself was in a state of crisis through a combination of overcrowding, escape attempts and disturbances. Those who wished to join the PMS were offered a career of 'great interest and importance' both in relation to the physical and psychological health of prisoners (*ibid.*: 104). The doctor's responsibilities included examining every prisoner on reception, visiting sick prisoners daily and dealing with questions of hygiene, sanitation, food, work and exercise for those prisoners 'undergoing certain forms of punishment or under mechanical restraint' (*ibid.*: 105). At the same time the importance of the psychiatric component in the work of the doctors was consistently underlined in the Prison Commissioners'

Reports. By the mid-1940s prisoners were broken down and placed into particular categories for psychiatric examination. This categorization was legitimated formally through the passing of the 1948 Criminal Justice Act which was an important moment in the post-war reconstruction of the criminal justice system.

The Act contained a number of important psychiatric provisions: courts were to consider the suitability reports submitted by the prison authorities on the mental and physical health of prisoners; it introduced two new psychiatric sentences which involved prison doctors in further diagnostic work; it allowed for the psychiatric training of prison hospital officers and the appointment of psychiatric social workers and prison psychologists who sat on the boards which determined whether prisoners were to be sent to open or closed prisons. From reports written by prison doctors at the time it is clear that the passing of the 1948 Act increased both their workload and their influence in the pre- and post-sentence stages. At the same time the psychiatric perspective articulated by many doctors did not find ready acceptance within the system. There were two principal reasons for this. First, the disciplinary direction of the prisons meant that those state servants who worked on the ground level – the prison officers – were highly sceptical about its ability to deliver the criminal. Indeed for many psychiatry was seen as an easy option which was likely to encourage the criminal rather than deter him or her. Second, prisoners themselves were highly sceptical about the benefits of psychological discourse. Immediately after the passing of the 1948 Act prison doctors and psychologists complained about the resistance of prisoners to their theories and the tendency of the confined to break off treatment.

Despite these critiques the role of medical power inside was still one which contained a strong disciplinary element. Within prison psychology there was increasing support for electroconvulsive therapy which itself was part of the tendency to individualize and medicalize deviance. This was also manifested through the use of leucotomies and the emergence of psychotropic drugs which by the late 1950s were receiving unqualified support from prison doctors as mechanisms of control (Sim 1990: 86–93). At the same time medical personnel were still involved in the disciplinary side of prison management and in setting out the required dietary provision for prisoners. Again, however, seen from the perspective of the confined their role was highly problematic. In 1948 Charles Carter edited the 28-page pamphlet *Snails Progress* which highlighted the experiences of Quaker prisoners between 1939 and 1948. Standards of hygiene and the conditions inside were often appalling with prisoners having to spend five weeks without a change of socks. The PMS was also a cause for concern, the medical inspection on admission was often trivial and the examination on discharge even more perfunctory, sometimes the newly admitted prisoner not even being required to undress (*The Lancet*, 31 July 1948: 191).

Gender and Prison Medicine

The relationship between confined women and the PMS has been almost totally neglected in academic work. And yet this relationship perhaps raises the starkest questions about standards of medical care inside and the role of medicine as a regulatory and disciplinary discourse. There are five issues that are important in relation to gender and prison medicine. First, male doctors had been heavily involved in judging women's behaviour and offering solutions to what they saw as deviant behaviour from the early nineteenth century. Once again their role became consolidated after 1895. Second, women were often seen as more intractable, violent and difficult than male prisoners and therefore needed particular forms of intervention to curb and control them. Third, the psychiatrization of women's behaviour which became institutionalized in the 1850s continued into the 1890s and beyond. Fourth, from 1885 penal institutions for women were headed by medical men who usually doubled as the prison governor. Although some women were appointed as governors after 1916 these women were also doctors (Sim 1990: 130–8). The final issue relates both to the question surrounding women's health care and to the particular mechanisms of control that were utilized to regulate the behaviour of confined women.

In terms of health care a number of accounts by prisoners and their supporters pointed to the often abysmal standards of attention that prisoners received. Florence Maybrick's description of medical services at Woking is one example of this (Maybrick 1905). The lack of medical treatment could have severe consequences. In May 1919 the Duchess of Bedford headed a Committee of Inquiry into the deaths of two prisoners in Holloway. One was Ellen Sullivan, a 17-year-old remandee who was continually vomiting and was 'attended by the wardresses on duty at the hospital, of whom not one was a trained nurse'. Before she died in the prison she gave birth to a child alone in her cell which lived for only a few minutes. The Prison Commissioners wrote to the governor of Holloway indicating that 'the section of the report dealing with verminous and dirty conditions should be carefully noted. It is evident that there has been a want of care and thought amounting to neglect in these matters' (cited in Sim 1990: 148). These sentiments were reinforced by the report of the Prison System Enquiry Committee which was published in 1922. It pointed to the poor standards of health care in general and the lack of attention paid to the special needs of women in relation to menstruation. In the same year Mary Gordon the first female inspector of prisons published her book *Penal Discipline* in which she pointed to: the lack of confidentiality between doctor and patient in prison; the fact that the doctor was a constable as well as a medical practitioner and that he was 'very much the heaviest hand over the prisoner in the affair of penal discipline' (Gordon 1922: 234–5). This 'heaviest hand' could pull doctors into areas where the ethical code around the protection of life was compromised. When Edith Thompson was executed in 1923 (for a crime of which she was innocent) the prison governor who was also the medical officer dealt with the prisoner's distraught protests by injecting her with drugs. The prisoner was then carried to the scaffold and propped up on the trap-door in order to fix the noose around her neck (Weis 1988: 301).

The question of medical care for women reverberated into the 1930s and 1940s. In 1943 the Prison Medical Reform Council published *Prisons for Women: Some Accounts of Life in Holloway.* The pamphlet pointed to: the superficial nature of the medical examination; the appalling conditions in which cleaning pails contained used sanitary towels; the fact that pregnant women were given the ordinary prison diet until they were six months pregnant and the ways in which doctors and nurses regarded the women as malingerers where illnesses were concerned or there was delay in receiving treatment (cited in Sim 1990: 156).

The issue around the delivery of health care for women was paralleled by the question of the role of medical staff in controlling and regulating the behaviour of confined women. In 1905 Florence Maybrick pointed to the involvement of prison doctors in the punishment of women: legitimating solitary confinement, bread and water diets, the use of straitjackets and the use of hobbles which was a particular instrument of punishment involving binding the wrists and ankles of the individual before strapping them behind her back. Prisoners' heads could also be shaved and blistered (Maybrick, *op. cit.*: 116–26). Suffragette women such as Constance Lytton also provided some chilling accounts of forced feeding. After a particularly horrendous episode she maintained that 'as the doctor left he gave me a slap on the cheek, not violently, but, as it were, to express his contemptuous disapproval, and he seemed to take for granted that my distress was assumed' (Lytton 1976: 268–70).

These particular forms of regulation and punishment for women offenders were underpinned by a broader set of discourses which became consolidated in the prison system in the twentieth century. These discourses were built around the psychiatrization of women's behaviour where prison doctors and increasingly psychologists attempted first to quantify the precise nature of women's deviance through psychological tests and second to normalize these women back to what was perceived as their 'natural role', i.e. a good wife and mother. Grace Pailthorpe's study in the 1930s was an important early example of this work. She concluded that female offenders were 'sick persons' who needed segregation and psychological correction:

> for women described as passive mental defectives, prone to promiscuity resulting in pregnancy, permanent segregation could be useful but sterilization would be best since it would allow them some freedom. (Dobash, Dobash and Gutteridge 1986: 121)

By the 1940s prison regimes were oriented to providing women with what the Prison Department reports described as 'a thorough grounding in mothercraft'. This was done by focusing on the psychological make-up of the 'neglectful mother' whose low intelligence was a manifestation of her abnormality and deviance. Consequently they were to be trained to be better housewives. The training was designed to instil into the women the ideals of a good home through stamping out their irresponsible behaviour. The positivist quantification of behaviour through psychological testing in the prison was thus a key element in this normalization process.

Conclusion

This paper has challenged the evolutionary model of medical history in prison. It has argued that prison doctors and psychologists did not stand outside or above the debates about crime and punishment between 1895 and 1948. Rather they were intimately involved in setting the parameters for the health care policies – both physical and psychological – which developed inside in those five decades. Despite differences between them and despite the humane services offered by individual doctors and psychologists, as a group prison health workers were united on an ideological terrain which was underpinned by discourses of discipline, individualization, regulation and medicalization. The power of medicine although challenged by prisoners and often resisted nonetheless became a potent force during these decades in the struggle to maintain not only the order of the prison but the wider social order itself. It is arguably a role which they have maintained up to the present historical moment.

References

M. Cousins and A. Hussain, *Michel Foucault* (Basingstoke: Macmillan, 1984).

R. Dobash, R. Dobash and S. Gutteridge, *The Imprisonment of Women* (Oxford: Blackwell, 1986).

M. Foucault, *Discipline and Punish* (Harmondsworth: Penguin, 1977)

D. Garland, *Punishment and Welfare* (Aldershot: Gower, 1985)

V. Gatrell, 'The Decline of Theft and Violence in Victorian and Edwardian England', in V. Gatrell, B. Lenman and G. Parker (eds), *Crime and the Law* (London: Europa, 1980), 238–337.

S. Hobhouse and F. Brockway, *English Prisons Today* (London: Longmans, Green and Co., 1922).

The Lancet, 30 March 1895.

The Lancet, 12 October 1895.

The Lancet, 31 July 1948.

C. Lytton, *Prisons and Prisoners: Experiences of a Suffragette* (Wakefield: E.P. Publishing, 1976).

W. Macartney, *Walls Have Mouths* (London: Victor Gollancz, 1936).

F. Maybrick, *Mrs Maybrick's Own Story: My Fifteen Lost Years* (London: Funk and Wagnalls Company, 1905).

S. O'Malley and G. Hall, 'I Have No Past', unpublished paper, 1988.

P. Patton, 'Of Power and Prisons', in M. Morris and P. Patton (eds), *Michel Foucault: Power, Truth and Strategy* (London: Ferrall, 1979), 109–47.

Prison Commissioners, *Statement By the Prison Commissioners of the Action Which Has Been Taken up to January 1898 to Carry Out the Recommendations in the Report of the Departmental Committee on Prisons 1895* (London: HMSO, 1898).

Prison Medical Reform Council, *Prison Medical Service* (London: Prison Medical Reform Council, 1943a).

Prison Medical Reform Council, *Prisoner's Circle* (London: Prison Medical Reform Council, 1943b).

Red Collar Man, *Chokey* (London: Victor Gollancz, 1937).

J. Sim, *Ordering for Care and Caring for Order* (Milton Keynes: unpublished Ph.D. thesis, The Open University, 1989).

J. Sim, *Medical Power in Prisons* (Milton Keynes: Open University Press, 1990).

S. Watson, *The Moral Imbecile: A Study of the Relations Between Penal Practice and Psychiatric Knowledge of the Habitual Offender* (Lancaster: unpublished Ph.D. thesis, University of Lancaster, 1988).

R. Weis, *Criminal Justice: The True Story of Edith Thompson* (London:

Hamish Hamilton, 1988).
M. Wiener, *Reconstructing the Criminal* (Cambridge: Cambridge University Press, 1990).
P. Young, 'Sociology, the state and penal relations', in D. Garland and P. Young (eds), *The Power to Punish* (London: Heinemann, 1983), 84–100.

Commentary

Dr Elizabeth Willis One question suggested from the title of Joe Sim's paper: I wondered if any data had been collected on the fate of the more consciously political deviant.

Sim There is some very interesting material from the 19th century which raises a series of questions about the specific treatment that the Irish prisoners received, and the codes of discipline, which were not utilized with regard to other prisoners. There is the argument about the 20th century in terms of the suffragettes and the types of medical treatment that those individuals received, with some very interesting parallels to be drawn there. More recently there are a number of biographical accounts of Irish prisoners in English jails in the 1970s and 1980s, but there has been no systematic study.

Porter Just to remind people that history does go back more than 150 years or so: there is a reasonable amount of evidence for a disproportionate severity of the legal system upon people with strong political views or people who are racially conspicuous. Peter Linebaug's excellent book *The London Hanged* dealing with the 18th and early 19th century suggests that the Irish, the Jews and black slaves etc. were punished more severely. Such people never got into the prisons, they got hanged. And this is not a frivolous point because there was a very ambiguous alliance between the justice system and the medical system in previous centuries, in that the only corpses that were legally available for dissection by the medical profession up to the early 19th century were those of executed felons: so there is a peculiar and sometimes rather sinister way in which the medical profession had an interest in the product of the justice system. And of course Hogarth brings it out peculiarly well in the last image in the "Four Stages of Cruelty' where you see the infamous hero or anti-hero actually being dissected by the Company of Surgeons. And the question which Hogarth is posing is: who is the crueller, the murderer whom you have seen through the sequence, or the surgeons who are dissecting his body?

Mrs K. W. Spencer-Lewis My research has led to the subject of peoples of African descent in relation to the Poor Laws and the tradition of racial discrimination with the importation of personal servants from the Commonwealth and colonies, and my question refers to information on people of African descent in prison institutions.

Sim I did not find information in relation to race either in the Public Record Office, or in the *British Medical Journal*, which were some of my main sources. That is not to say that it is not there. I am about to make a study of sources from Walton Prison and I would expect to find material relating to prisoners of African descent.

Summers Can anybody here suggest the earliest date when chemical means were used for restraint of refractory prisoners, as opposed to strait-jackets, dark cells, ankle straps and the like?

Sim The twentieth-century use of psychotropic agents has a long history which includes other medical methods: there is a record of a form of electro-convulsive therapy used on a female prisoner as long ago as 1811.

7

Prison Doctors and Prison Suicide Research

Alison Liebling and Tony Ward

An intensely controversial question is being asked at the moment behind the doors of Prison Service headquarters: if, as seems likely, prison suicide is not exclusively or even largely a psychiatric problem, why should prison doctors have such a disproportionate amount of power and responsibility in the prevention, management and diagnosis of suicide risk? Some prison doctors are beginning to want to relinquish some of this power and to share it with others. But after decades of mounting criticism of prisons in the wake of increasing numbers of prison suicides, few of their colleagues are eager to share the power and responsibility with them.

In the search for a clearer understanding of both suicide and the organization of its management and prevention, it became increasingly important to find out whether our current inheritance came about by design or by accident of history. The legacy of this history in contemporary prison life is illustrated by the question Alison Liebling was asked when she embarked on what turned out to be five years of research on prison suicide: 'But you're not a doctor! You must be a psychiatrist, then?' This inadequacy was rectified by the appointment of a psychiatrist as her Ph.D. supervisor and the insistence that at least one of the external examiners be a psychiatrist. As it happened, the psychiatrist appointed as external examiner was the same one who, years before, had pointed out to his student that prison suicide wasn't a psychiatric problem, but a management problem (see Scottish Home and Health Department, 1985). This acknowledgement has only recently been translated into policy (see Home Office, 1992).

Why, then, has the problem always been studied and managed by the medical profession? In this paper we concentrate on the research aspect of the medical role. We shall first summarize the findings of the earliest pieces of research into prison suicide in England and Wales, and then offer a more critical reading of two of the studies which situates their explanations of suicide in the context of the penal discourses of their times.

Early Studies of Prison Suicide

It comes as no surprise to discover that the first three substantial studies of prison suicide in England and Wales were carried out by prison doctors (Gover, 1879; Smalley, 1911; Topp, 1979). What is perhaps more surprising is that the first two studies do not define the problem in such a way as to suggest that suicide prevention is primarily a medical responsibility. Both these studies are to be found in the Prison Commissioners' annual reports. Their authors wrote as Medical Inspectors of Prisons, whose contributions to the annual reports always included some discussion of mortality statistics. Prison suicide fell within the scope of medical knowledge simply by virtue of being a mode of death, whether or not any psychiatric factor was involved.

The first study, by Dr R.M. Gover, was based on responses to a questionnaire circulated by the Prison Commissioners to the governors, medical officers and chaplains of local prisons in 1879. The Commissioners had assumed responsibility for the local prisons in 1878, and their investigation was prompted by the fact that the suicide rate in the local prisons appeared to be some four times as high as that in the convict prisons (Commissioners of Prisons, 1879: 16–17; Gover, 1879: 54).

Dr Gover concluded from his survey of 81 suicides in local prisons over the five and a half years up to 31 March 1879 that suicides occurred most frequently during the first week of custody. He observed that those most vulnerable to suicide were first-time prisoners (42 per cent of the suicides had no previous convictions recorded against them) and those on remand (34 per cent of the suicides). Suspense and anxiety relating to the trial were put forward as a possible explanation. Other groups particularly prone to suicide were prisoners convicted of violent offences, those anticipating penal servitude, and those awaiting trial to a convict prison, having already received a sentence of penal servitude. An analysis of the occupation of those ending their lives in this way showed that most were mechanics or labourers. Fear – of penal servitude, but also of other fates – was the most influential of the motives for suicide. Gover suggested that prison staff's lack of knowledge of individual prisoners was a relevant factor. Those prisons whose governors and chaplains were least able to assign motives to the suicides were those where the largest number of suicides occurred.

Gover concluded that in prison, the operation of 'a principle analogous to the survival of the fittest' could be detected, 'the most hardened criminals being those best able to endure imprisonment' (p. 59): the most often imprisoned were not the most at risk.

Sir Herbert Smalley, Gover's successor, analysed those suicides occurring between 1902 and 1911 (Smalley, 1911). He found that there was an average of 9.5 suicides per annum (range 4–14). The total number for the whole period was 95 (86 males and 9 females). Smalley noted that 'the number of females, nine, is too small for statistical analysis'; they were therefore excluded from the rest of the study. Despite the fact that Norwich Prison was at that time 'haunted' by a female prisoner suicide who was known to stalk the corridors at night, suicide by women prisoners has received very little treatment in official reports, then or now (see Liebling, 1993). Smalley argued that the most striking difference between suicides in prison and ordinary suicides was in respect of their age: the incidence of suicide in prison was much higher in the younger age-groups. Outside, it was known that suicides occurred more frequently among the older age-groups: at least 55 per cent of male suicides were aged over 45 (Smalley, 1911: 41). Of the 86 male prison suicides in his study, 6 were under 30 years old, 19 were aged between 20 and 24; 22 were aged 25–34; 18 aged 35–44; and only 21 (24.4 per cent) were aged 45 or over. This difference in age distribution between suicides in and out of prison could not be accounted for by the uneven age distribution of the prison population alone. 'It is probable, therefore', Smalley concluded, 'that some other influences are operative either in the special character of persons going to prison or in the special conditions that attach to imprisonment' (p. 41).

Forty-three (50 per cent) of Smalley's male suicides had been imprisoned for acquisitive crimes; 12 (41 per cent) for homicide (murder, manslaughter and wounding with intent to murder); four for sexual offences (carnal knowledge, rape and sodomy); three for indecent exposure; four each for arson, vagrancy and drunkenness; one for wilful damage; and one for brothel-keeping. Three had been imprisoned for attempted suicide: between 1909 and 1913, about 2,400 people a year were arrested for this offence, of whom 28 per cent received prison sentences (Anderson, 1987: 288, 303). Offenders convicted of impulsive violence or crimes against morality (sexual offences) were found to be most 'prone to suicide': for example, 14 per cent of prison suicides were imprisoned for homicide offences, yet such offenders accounted for only 2.4 per cent of the prison population (p. 41). Crimes of arson were also over-represented amongst prison suicides.

Smalley commented that suicidal tendency appeared in most cases to be related to the nature of the offence and not to the anticipated severity of the punishment facing the prisoner, except perhaps in offences of exceptional gravity. He argued that although insanity was frequently associated with violent crimes:

> It is not, however, to be assumed from this that suicide is in such cases necessarily the result of insanity. It is quite probable that in many instances an impulsive suicide, like the impulsive crime which preceded it, may be an initial symptom of mental disease, but in the absence of other evidence it is at least as likely that the emotional instability shown in the crime and in the suicide may be due to conditions within the limits of mental health. This is notably the case, for instance, in children and adolescents; and the earlier age incidence in prison suicides ... may perhaps be taken to point to the physiological instability of youth as shown by impulsive reaction to the shock of detection or of imprisonment. (p. 41)

Two other studies from this period touched on the question of prison suicide, though it was not their main concern. Both the alienist and barrister S.A.K. Strahan in *Suicide and Insanity* (1893: 103–4) and the prison doctor Charles Goring in *The English Convict* (1913: 152–3) observed that suicide accounted for a much higher proportion of deaths in prison than of deaths in the community. This was an unfortunate choice of base rate, as suicides as a proportion of deaths are not an indication of suicide rates. Strahan found that from 1879 to 1891, suicide was 'about twenty-four times more commonly a cause of death among those who die in our prisons than among those who die outside them, [even] after the insane are winnowed from their ranks' by being transferred to asylums (p. 104). Although 'disgrace, remorse and black despair' might account for some suicides, the main factor in Strahan's view was the 'innate degeneracy' of the prison population. Goring, on the other hand, explained the pattern of deaths by the environmental conditions of English prisons, and noted that 'the special immunity from accidental death, afforded to prisoners, happens to be nicely balanced by their increased liability to die from suicide' (Goring, 1913: 153).

Although these four writers differed over the importance to be attached to the prison environment and to the innate characteristics of prisoners, none of them attempted to construct a profile of a suicide-prone *individual.* Their analyses were limited to demonstrating and explaining the relatively high suicide rates of the prison population as a whole, or of particular demographic or legal categories within it. Where 'physiological' factors such as 'degeneracy' were invoked, they were characteristics which suicidal prisoners were assumed to share with other offenders of a similar kind. There were, however, some noteworthy differences between Gover's and Smalley's analyses of suicide rates (these being the only two which are detailed enough to repay examination in depth), and these reflected important changes in penal policy and in the doctor's role within it.

Gover: Fear, Shame and Deterrence

Gover was writing in the early years of the centralized prison service, under the directorship of Sir Edmund DuCane. The chief aim of the prison system was general deterrence, the chief means of achieving it was the bureaucratic enforcement of a uniform set of rules (Radzinowicz and Hood, 1986: 628–9; Forsythe, 1987: 193–214). As Sim (1990: 50–1) has shown, one of the functions of prison doctors was to assist in the formulation of rules that would achieve the maximum deterrent effect without permanently damaging the prisoner's health (see also Wiener, this volume). Prison deaths were politically sensitive because they suggested that the authorities had got the balance wrong (Sim and Ward, 1994). Although deaths linked to an allegedly inadequate diet figured especially prominently in this debate, critics such as *The Lancet* also pointed to suicides as a product of an excessively harsh and uniform regime (*Lancet*, 1887, cited by Sim, 1990: 51). Another critic who took this view was Henry Harcourt, whose evidence to the Royal Commission on Penal Servitude was based on his own experience as a prisoner. Harcourt had been at Millbank when Gover was medical officer there, and his comments on the doctor, as Anne Hardy (this volume) remarks, were generally very favourable. He described one incident, however, when a prisoner was 'carried into the infirmary almost in dying state; he was a boy. I was then a nurse in the infirmary. I heard Dr Gover say, "Well, I will put mustard plaster and such as that to him;" and he said to him, "I have a good mind to have you flogged; if you attempt it again I will have you flogged."' (Royal Commission, 1878, Q. 4393)

Harcourt went on to suggest that there were many reasons for a prisoner to contemplate suicide: 'In the case of a man who has never been in prison before, there is the shock of entering prison, then again there is the walking round and round the yard at such a distance apart, and with no-one to communicate or converse with you; then there is continually having the officer spy on you through a little slit in your wall, and brutal officers coming to you, and if your back is tired after sitting in one position (you have nothing else than a bucket of water with a piece of board on top to sit upon at Millbank) and you move your bucket closer to the wall, to rest your back against it, you are reported for it.' (Q. 4440)

Gover, not surprisingly, interpreted his findings in such a way as to refute any suggestion that the cruelty of the prison regime was responsible for suicide. He pointed to the finding that 66 of the 81 prisoners who killed themselves had never been punished for any disciplinary offence as showing that 'such mental depression and physical discomfort as may result from the infliction of punishments for breaches of prison discipline has but little effect in inducing attempts at suicide' (p. 60). Commenting on the finding that suicide was commonest in the early stages of a sentence, he remarked: 'Possibly a prolonged acquaintance with the interior of a modern prison may in many cases have the effect of quieting apprehensions and depriving imprisonment of imaginary terrors' (p. 58). He noted that the crimes committed by suicidal prisoners were not, for the most part, 'likely to be committed by persons of education', a fact which 'so far as it goes, tends to indicate that such persons tolerate imprisonment better than is generally supposed' (p. 60). Gover also pointed out that whilst the fear of being sent to a convict prison was the commonest motive assigned for suicide, the actual rate of suicide in those prisons was relatively low: 'The only explanation for these figures would appear to be that penal servitude is much dreaded, by reason of its effect upon the imagination, while the fears which it inspires are not found to be justified by actual experience' (p. 59). That penal servitude should inspire fear was, of course, just as it should be. Gover called particular attention to the finding that nine prisoners who showed 'no marked indications of depression ... deliberately preferred death to being sent to a convict prison' (p. 61) – a vivid indication of the effectiveness of the prison in striking terror into the heart of the criminal.

We have noted that Gover, unlike many later researchers, made some attempt to ascertain prisoners' motives for killing themselves. He explained that 'The Commissioners decided to avail themselves as far as possible of the knowledge possessed by governors and chaplains of the character and disposition of prisoners individually, by including in the circular a question as to the "supposed motive"' (p. 60). In fact the same question was asked of medical officers (p. 56) but Gover provided no information as to their responses, and he criticized only the governors and chaplains who, 'in nearly half the cases', replied that the motive was 'not known' (p. 60). We may suppose that Gover was not anxious to criticize his professional colleagues, but also that he did not consider a knowledge of suicidal motivation to be chiefly the province of the medical officer.

At this time it was primarily the chaplain, rather than the doctor, who would be expected to have some knowledge of individual prisoners' states of mind (Walker and McCabe, 1973: 50–1). The chaplain also had some claim to expertise on the subject of suicidal motivation, particularly on account of his role in dealing with prisoners charged with attempted suicide. 'In so far as mid-Victorian London ever had a suicide prevention agency', writes Anderson (1987: 317), 'it was surely located in the chaplain's office in Clerkenwell', London's main remand prison. Clerkenwell's chaplain, John Horsley, certainly considered himself an expert on suicide: 'I suppose that no-one in the world has similar or as great opportunities of observing the phenomena of this particular crime', he told readers of *The Fortnightly* in 1881 (quoted by Anderson, 1987: 327). His ideas on motivation (as paraphrased by Anderson, p. 320) were straightforward: 'Suicide, like every other kind of sin, crime and misery, was caused by intemperance, impurity, laziness, and bad temper, and nothing else.'

The two motives highlighted by Gover on the basis of the chaplain's and governor's reports were 'fear' and 'shame'. The fact that nine suicides were ascribed to 'shame' and only two to 'remorse' seemed to Gover to confirm 'the truth of the common saying that men do not suffer so much from consciousness of guilt as from the consequences of discovery' (pp. 61–2). The *naïveté* of this reasoning – using the fact that motives ascribed by officials reflect conventional wisdom to confirm that conventional wisdom is true – might seem obvious, but contemporary suicidologists have little right to be condescending on this score. Similar but slightly more subtle forms of circular reasoning, by which researchers accept definitions of suicide based on coroners' and other officials' assumptions about what suicide 'looks like', are endemic in studies of suicide in general and prison suicide in particular. Sociological critiques of this process (Douglas, 1967; Atkinson, 1978; Taylor, 1982) seem to have made little impression on prison suicide research (Liebling, 1992: 85–6).

Prisoners' mental states would, of course, come within the purview of the medical officer where there was a suspicion that their minds were 'unsound'. Findings of insanity were not made lightly, and the prison medical officer had to be wary of malingerers who would feign insanity, and even attempted suicide, in order to escape the full rigours of the prison regime (Saunders, 1981, 1988; Royal Commission, 1878). Only two suicidal prisoners were considered to have been of unsound mind, even though 'in nearly every instance of suicide in prison the verdict of the coroner's jury is "committed suicide while in a state of temporary insanity"'(p. 62).

Coroners' juries at this time were often critical of prisons and particularly of their medical officers (Sim and Ward, 1994). Although inquests frequently (but by no means invariably) found suicides 'temporarily insane', thus absolving them from criminal responsibility for their deaths, and allowing their families to benefit from any life-insurance they had (Anderson, 1987: 218–28), in the case of prisoners (who were unlikely to have insured their lives and could hardly be spared the stigma of criminality) such a verdict could well be seen as implied criticism of the prison – what, after all, was likely to have driven them temporarily insane?

Gover suggested that had governors and chaplains known more about motives for suicide they might have been able to take precautions against it. It is quite unclear, however, how governors or chaplains were supposed to acquire a detailed knowledge of individual motivation in prisons such as Strangeways (daily average population 899), Preston (527) and Wakefield (1,201). (On the infrequency of chaplains' visits to individual prisoners see McConville, 1981: 446–7; Priestly, 1981: 113.) There is a certain irony in these three large establishments being singled out for their high suicide rates, with the implication that poor management by the governor and chaplain was somehow to blame, since Gover also made the point that the overall death rate (including natural deaths) was highest in the smallest establishments, due in part to the 'superior organisation of large prisons' (p. 54). Both the high death rate in small prisons, and the high suicide rate in local prisons generally, seem to be taken as indications that there is scope for the new Prison Commission to improve local management; or in the case of small prisons, to reduce the death rate by closing them (Commissioners of Prisons, 1879: 17, 54).

Smalley: Adolescence, Impulsiveness and Reformation

The period between Gover's report and Smalley's witnessed a fundamental transformation in English penal discourse (Garland, 1985). General deterrence and rigid uniformity, the hallmarks of the late Victorian penal system, had by Smalley's time given way – at least in theory – to rehabilitation and individualization. The Probation of Offenders Act 1907 and the Prevention of Crime Act 1908 had placed probation and Borstal training, respectively, on a statutory footing, and Home Office officials were committed to reducing the prison population (Rutherford, 1986: 124).

Within the prisons, the importance of the medical officers had grown as that of the chaplains had declined. After 1889 an increasing part of their work was the preparation of reports on 'doubtful cases' of insanity (Walker and McCabe, 1971: 59) and they were building up a body of expertise on the causes of suicide, a fertile area for the investigation of 'one of the most discussed questions of the day, namely, the links between deviant behaviour, degeneracy, insanity, feeble-mindedness and inebriety' (Anderson, 1987: 391). Contemporaneously with Smalley's report, his colleague W. Norwood East was working on a major study of 1,000 attempted suicides. (East (1913) did not specifically discuss prison suicides, but his finding (p. 468) that arrests for offences against the person were more often followed by suicide attempts than those for property offences was consistent with Smalley's.)

Despite the different context in which he was writing, Smalley's analysis was in some respects strikingly similar to Gover's. He pointed to the high incidence of suicide in the first week of imprisonment, and its rarity in convict prisons, as evidence that 'imprisonment, *per se*, is not an inducement to self destruction' (p. 42), although the 'shock of detection or of imprisonment' might be (p. 41). He also pointed to an association between suicide and certain crimes (homicide, arson and sexual offences) as evidence that there was some common characteristic of the individual which led to both crime and suicide. For Gover the common factor was a 'constitutional' predisposition to violence; for Smalley it was 'impulsiveness' (p. 41).

As we have seen, Smalley argued that such 'impulsiveness', though it might sometimes be an early symptom of insanity, could also arise from 'emotional instability ... due to conditions within the limits of mental health' (p. 41). Such conditions were not necessarily beyond the limits of medical interest. The idea that forms of mental instability falling short of insanity contributed both to crime and to problems of discipline was espoused by many prison doctors at this time, and was an area in which they could claim special expertise (Watson, 1988). Smalley had made a significant contribution to this debate, highlighting in particular the problems posed by 'feeble-minded' prisoners (Sim, 1990: 66–7) who were shortly to be catered for by the Mental Defectives Act 1913. In his report for 1903–4, Smalley singled out 'chronic alcoholics and epileptics' – two of the main categories of 'weak-minded' prisoners – as especially prone to act on sudden (and unpredictable) suicidal impulses (Smalley, 1905: 40).

In 1911, however, Smalley shifted his focus to 'children and adolescents' as being especially prone to 'emotional instability', and hence to suicide, due to the influence of the 'physiological instability of youth' (p. 41). The 'adolescent', whose 'physiological instability' gave rise to emotional impulsiveness and delinquency, had emerged as a distinct and problematic social category around the turn of the century (Bailey, 1987: 8–9; Clarke, 1985: 240–1). Smalley, a strong advocate of the new Borstal system, applied his interest in biometrics (Anderson, 1987: 391) to a study of the heights and weights of young offenders at various ages, seeking to demonstrate that their 'inferiority of organization' was largely attributable to environmental factors 'affecting development during those years of adolescence which, as we know, are also the formative period of the criminal habit and the criminal character' (Smalley, 1908: 480). Borstal training, for Smalley, was the ideal corrective for both the moral and physical effects of an 'evil environment'. In his 1911 report, he emphasized 'the need for exercising discretion in inflicting imprisonment on young offenders, and desirability of making the treatment of such offenders educative and reformatory rather than merely punitive' as 'highly important' for suicide prevention (pp. 41–2). Indeed this was his only recommendation. Thus the suicide statistics turn out to be a vindication of the rehabilitationist and reductionist penal policies of Smalley's time, just as Gover's findings were a vindication of the deterrent regime of the Victorian penitentiary.

Smalley's report coincided with the opening of a second Borstal institution at Feltham, in response to lobbying from magistrates and judges who wanted the scheme extended to those who were being rejected by the Prison Commissioners as mentally or physically unfit for the existing institution at Borstal, Kent (Radzinowicz and Hood, 1986: 389–90). Feltham has remained one of the main centres for young offenders with psychiatric problems. Its 'educative and reformatory' regime could well have been just what Smalley had in mind to alleviate the problems of suicidal young prisoners. If so, it is a sad irony that four of Feltham's young prisoners took their own lives in 1991–2 (Howard League, 1993).

Research and Prevention

Despite the changes in penal strategies between Gover's time and Smalley's, and between Smalley's and our own, strategies for the prevention of suicide seem to have changed remarkably little. In 1878 the Chief Surgeon of the convict prison at Pentonville described how a prisoner who showed signs of suicidal tendencies would be 'sent to a cell called a medical observation cell, the trap door of which kept constantly open, and certain directions are given to the officers that this prisoner is to be specially watched.... The furniture of his cell is always removed.... His bed is replaced at night, but he is deprived of his braces and other things with which he is likely to suspend himself.' (Royal Commission, 1878–9, Qq. 1924–6)

Smalley, in his report for 1903–4, described how in local prisons,

> Every care is taken when there are reasonable suspicions of a suicidal tendency to deprive prisoners of any facility for carrying out their intentions, either by placing them under special observation, when they are visited frequently by an officer, in association with other prisoners under close and continuous observation of an officer, or even by detailing officers to watch over them day and night. (Smalley, 1904: 41)

In modern terminology, these are descriptions to the 'strip cell' and the different varieties of 'special watch', which have remained the mainstays of suicide prevention in prisons until the present day (although, at the level of policy at least, important changes in official thinking about suicide prevention are now under way). In the early years of this century, Smalley was already pointing out the inherent limitations of this approach: 'excessive surveillance' could 'become irksome to the individual while entailing ... unnecessary expense' (Smalley, 1904: 41) and in any case suicide was unpredictable and not the prerogative of any clinically definable category of prisoner. In Smalley's 1911 report the prevention of suicide, among young prisoners at least, was explicitly linked with reduction in the use of custody and with reform of custodial regimes. Sadly, the crude preventive techniques of Smalley's day seem to have had a more lasting influence than the broader approach to prevention suggested by his research.

References

Anderson, O., *Suicide in Victorian and Edwardian England* (Oxford: Clarendon Press, 1987).

Atkinson, J.M., *Discovering Suicide* (London: Macmillan, 1978).

Bailey, V., *Delinquency and Citizenship* (Oxford: Clarendon Press, 1987).

Clarke, J., 'Managing the delinquent', in M. Langan and B. Schwartz (eds), *Crises in the British State, 1880–1930* (London: Hutchinson, 1985).

Commissioners of Prisons, *Annual Report 1878–9, PP* (1878–9) xxxiv, 1.

Douglas, J., *The Social Meanings of Suicide* (London: Routledge, 1967).

East, W.N., 'On attempted suicide, with an analysis of 1,000 consecutive cases', *Journal of Mental Science*, 59 (1913), 428–78.

Forsythe, W.J., *The Reform of Prisoners, 1830–1900* (London: Croom Helm, 1987).

Garland, D., *Punishment and Welfare* (Aldershot: Gower, 1985).
Gover, R.M., 'Notes by the Medical Inspector', in Commissioners of Prisons (1879).
Home Office, *The Way Forward: Caring for Prisoners at Risk of Suicide and Self-Injury*, information paper issued by DIA 1 (London, 1992).
Howard League *Suicides in Feltham* (London: author, 1993).
Liebling, A., *Suicides in Prison* (London: Routledge, 1992).
Liebling, A., 'Suicide Amongst Women Prisoners', *Howard Journal*, 33 (1994), 1–9.
McConville. S., *A History of English Prison Administration. Volume 1: 1750–1887* (London: Routledge, 1981).
Priestly, P., *Victorian Prison Lives* (London: Methuen, 1985).
Royal Commission on Penal Servitude, *Report, Parliamentary Papers* (1878) xxxvii, 1.
Rutherford, A., *Prisons and the Process of Justice* (Oxford: Oxford University Press, 1986).
Saunders, J., 'Magistrates and madmen', in V. Bailey (ed.), *Policing and Punishment in the Nineteenth Century* (London: Croom Helm, 1981).
Saunders, J., 'Quarantining the weak-minded', in W. F. Bynum, R. Porter and M. Shepherd (eds), *The Anatomy of Madness*, vol. 3 (London: Tavistock, 1988).
Scottish Home and Health Department, *Report on a Review of Suicide Prevention at HM Detention Centre and Young Offenders Institution, Glenochil* (Edinburgh: HMSO, 1985).
Sim, J., *Medical Power in Prisons* (Buckingham: Open University Press, 1990).
Sim, J. and Ward, T., 'The magistrate of the poor? Coroners and deaths in custody in nineteenth century England', in M. J. Clarke and C. Crawford (eds), *Legal Medicine in History* (Cambridge: Cambridge University Press 1994).
Smalley, H., 'Report by the Medical Inspector', in Commissioners of Prisons, *Annual Report for 1903–4, PP* (1905) xxxvii, 40–2.
Smalley, H., 'Report by the Medical Inspector', in Commissioners of Prisons, *Annual Report for 1907–8, PP* (1908) lii, 478–80.
Smalley, H., 'Report by the Medical Inspector', in Commissioners of Prisons, *Annual Report for 1910–11, PP* (1911) xxxix, 243.
Taylor, S., *Durkheim and the Study of Suicide* (London: Macmillan, 1982).
Topp, D. O., 'Suicide in British prisons', *British Journal of Psychiatry*, 134 (1979), 24–7.
Walker, N. and McCabe, S., *Crime and Insanity in England*, vol. 2 (Edinburgh: Edinburgh University Press, 1971).
Watson, S., *The Moral Imbecile*, unpublished Ph.D. thesis, University of Lancaster.

Commentary

Liebling (In response to a question) My mission has been to teach those who do not work in prisons that the staff are charged with looking after an extremely vulnerable population. The suicide rate amongst young males has gone up quite drastically in the last 10–15 years, and as we have increased our efforts to keep young offenders out of prison the population that remains behind the walls are a selected and vulnerable group. That means that part of the increase in the rate of suicide in prison can be explained by the increase in the rate outside, and the increase has been almost confined to the lower social groups. It has been shown by a study in Edinburgh that suicide occurs very selectively amongst the young, and we also imprison very selectively, so it is arguable whether what we have inside is a reflection of what we have outside. People use the term 'attention-seeking behaviour': it is probably fairer to say that delinquent behaviour is often amongst adolescents an expression of serious problems of depression. Acting out feelings in behaviour is a characteristic of adolescence which they are likely to bring into imprisonment with them: they are then exposed to an environment which many of them find they just cannot deal with.

Ward (In response to a question) We have a figure for how many were in for attempted suicide when this was a criminal offence. In Smalley's sample 3 out of 86 suicides were in prison for attempted suicide.

Ward (In response to a question) Smalley commented on the methods of close surveillance in use in an attempt to prevent suicide in prison and pointed out its limitations. Excessive surveillance could be irksome for the individual and also expensive and it was difficult to know whom to observe.

Liebling From the point of view of prison staff only 30% of completed suicides in prison have had any contact with psychiatric services: they do not have a psychiatric illness. When you take the young this decreases to something like 13%: so in 87% of prison suicides for the young 'under 21' there is no psychiatric diagnosis that can be made. A common sequence – although things are changing – is that a prison officer who thinks that he might have a suicidal prisoner on his hands refers to a psychiatric specialist who reports no psychiatric illness, and sends him back from hospital to the wing. The prison officer may conclude that his concerns are needless and the prisoner is then found hanged. Prison officers have believed that psychiatrists are the only kind of people who have any knowledge or understanding about prison suicide, and that they are the only people to have an opinion that counts, both in practice and in theoretical understanding of the problem. That inheritance is a problem. Why do prison officers resist their own intuitive understanding about suicide risk? That is why psychiatrists have retained legislative control.

Liebling (In response to a question) There have been some studies on prisoners recently released, and it has been shown, not in Britain but in other European countries, that in the year following release, young prisoners are four times more likely to die, from several causes: from suicide, from drug abuse, from road accidents and from other causes; and I would guess that they are equally at risk if they were on bail.

Dr Dorothy Black It does seem to me that the psychiatrist has some role to play in excluding people with serious depressive illness. Recent work in Cardiff Prison and elsewhere has been done to develop self-help groups where clearly identified and willing prisoners would act themselves as counsellors and monitors of younger prisoners. These people are in day-to-day contact with new juveniles and new adolescent prisoners coming into the prison. From the follow-up they seem to be more effective in preventing attempted suicide.

Speaker I refer to the Listener schemes which were pioneered in Swansea Prison after the death of Philip Knight who was 15 years old. That death upset staff and prisoners so much that there was a very radical working party – the first to have prisoners invited to talk about how to prevent suicides in prison. The team at Swansea was led by the Probation Service and it has been exported, with a lot of effort from staff and prisoners, to at least 30 other establishments in the country. They have been supported by the Samaritans, who come in and train selected volunteer prisoners to act as Samaritans to other prisoners; and one of the most important elements to feed into this scheme was the result of research which showed that if you talk to prisoners who have attempted suicide, they were the most sympathetic recipients. They would talk far more articulately about why prisoners attempted suicide than any other group, and were very distinct in the way they explained other prisoners' suicide, having been close to it often themselves.

Tumim Could I just add two points from my review on suicide (1990). It was a principal point that it was not just the psychiatrist or the doctor who should be the only person keeping an eye open for possible suicide: it is essential that the whole staff and other inmates take part in it, and not leave it to doctors, of one sort or another. That was a theme which went through the report and was, I think, accepted by ministers as desirable. The second thing, on a quite different point: the Listener schemes which are now being developed, not only in Swansea but elsewhere, are obviously of the highest value in putting forward these matters, and certainly as far as the Inspectorate are concerned we are glad to commend them where we find them, and do what we can to encourage some sort of scheme in which other inmates are involved in helping possible suicidal persons.

Smith Has there been an attempt to evaluate this scheme, which has been going on in some prisons and not in others?

Liebling Not yet.

Summers Could I add a historical note? The first thing Elizabeth Fry did in Newgate was to get the prisoners to elect their own monitors and school mistress. This development was condemned by the inspector.

Tumim I am against prefects and monitors in prisons and the Inspectorate continues to say the same.

Speaker Is the copy-cat effect a real thing?

Speaker Those of you who watch *East Enders* will recall that the woman who worked in the pub took an overdose: it was shown that in the weeks following the episode not only was there an increased number of over doses admitted to hospitals, but that it was particularly amongst a group which resembled the woman who took the overdose on the television programme – the same age and social background. The only good methodological studies have been carried out in the USA and they show that if you have a teenage suicide on television, particularly where a series has been repeated, it can be shown statistically that there is an increase amongst similar people, not just a disorganised (general) increase. Our establishments have a high concentration of very vulnerable prisoners, and when one prisoner takes his own life, then there are likely to be those who make the decision to cross a threshold and those effects have been shown in more than one establishment.

Tumim The onus of the Woolf Report is clear, that disturbances in prison are copied elsewhere, and Lord Woolf found after Manchester that groups felt they had to show they were macho by getting out on the roof: there was certainly a big copy-cat part in the April 1990 disturbances.

Dr Paul Knapman I wonder if I could say something. I am a coroner and we can't have it both ways. Every case of both natural and unnatural death that occurs in a prison has to be the subject of an inquest. It has to be in public and that has been the law for a very long time. Now that may well be the reason for the publicity and it could follow from that that there are copy-cat phenomena. The alternative of course is to hold such things in camera, but I suspect that there are a lot of people here who would think that that would be a very retrograde step. We must make our mind up: I cannot see a middle course. Every case comes before the Coroner's Court and is very likely to be reported.

8

Health Services for Prisoners: Lost in Ambiguities

Richard Smith

The recent history of prisons and prison health care in Britain is rich in rhetoric and bare in change in conditions for the average prisoner. I first became interested in prison health care in the early 1980s,[1] and since then we have had a major report from the Woolf Committee,[2] dozens of reports from the Chief Inspector of Prisons, and reports on health care from the House of Commons Social Services Committee[3] and the royal medical colleges;[4] and the Prison Medical Service has changed its name to the Health Service for Prisoners. Yet I doubt if most of the people in prison in 1980 who are still there would notice any change at all. British prisons remain squalid, brutal and overcrowded, and the health care of prisoners continues to be second rate. Britain has what are undoubtedly some of the worst prisons in the developed world.[5]

Much of this resistance to change stems from prisons being institutions that are geographically and socially isolated where every aspect of life is controlled. Most people in Britain have never been into a prison. Yet many of those who work in prisons have been doing so for a long time, and most of the prisoners are recurrent offenders. Politicians and senior administrators responsible for prisons come and go rapidly, but most of those inside the prisons remain. It's thus not surprising that prisons change little. In addition, political anxieties over prisons may be largely discharged by words. To develop the rhetoric into real change may be politically risky.

Another reason, I believe, for the slowness of change is the lack of a clear mission in the prison service. We are not clear what prisons are for, and ideas on the purposes of imprisonment have changed over time. The theories on change management produced by management theorists suggest that a clear mission and strategy are essential for successful change. Effective organizations know why they exist and what they are trying to achieve. The leaders of the organization spread the mission through the organization so that people understand the mission and subscribe to it. Only then can the organization achieve its aims and change effectively.

My argument in this paper is that we are not clear what prisons are for. A consequence of this, which I will explore, is that the prison medical service is confused in its role. This confusion stops it performing to the highest standard and creates many difficulties for the service when it tries to respond to the many problems it faces.

Although the prison service does not have a clear mission, it does have a mission statement. It reads: 'Her Majesty's Prison Service serves the public by keeping in custody those committed by the courts. Our duty is to look after them with humanity and to help them lead law abiding and useful lives in custody and after release.' As with most mission statements, much thought is collapsed into these bland words. There is just a hint of the possibility that prisons might lead inmates to better lives, but the statement begins with the assertion that the first job of prisons is to serve the courts. This is the usual answer from those working in prisons to the question 'What are prisons for?' The implication is that it is not for prison employees to tell courts that they are sending too many or the wrong people to prison. If the courts want to send more people to prison than the prisons can accommodate then the prison service must cram several prisoners into each cell or open army camps to take the overflow. Similarly it is no function of the courts or the judiciary to consider the difficulties of the prisons when deciding whether or not to sentence somebody to imprisonment. The problem with this separation between the courts and the prisons is that it makes for overcrowding and poor management.

The purpose of imprisonment in the minds of most members of the public is punishment. Every so often there is an outcry in the press about prisoners living in 'soft' conditions, and many members of the public think that living in poor conditions in prison is part of the punishment. Yet ever since the Gladstone Committee of 1895 people are supposedly sent to prison 'as punishment' not 'for punishment'.[6] But the dreadful conditions in many prisons and the second-rate services mean in reality that prisoners suffer much more than removal of their liberty. There is thus confusion over this aim of imprisonment, and the confusion affects the medical services in that the authorities are willing to tolerate standards that would not be acceptable in the outside world. Second-class services would not be allowed if the authorities were serious that people were sent to prison as, not for, punishment.

Another aim of imprisonment is to protect the public by keeping dangerous people out of the way. The problem with even this simple aim is that few prisoners are really dangerous; and telling who exactly is dangerous is hard, even impossible. Probably no more than 5 per cent of prisoners are dangerous in the sense that they would be highly likely to commit violent crimes if released. The idea that a primary aim of imprisonment is protecting the public leads to an obsession with security, which constantly gets in the way of other activities – like health care or education.

Every so often the idea surfaces that prisons are there to deter prisoners from re-offending. Reconviction rates are a standard measure in criminology rather in the way that mortality rates are a standard measure in health care, and all the evidence is that those imprisoned are highly likely to be imprisoned again. Something like three-quarters of those released from prison will be sent back again. This is because prisoners learn more about the mechanics of crime (hence the phrase 'schools for recidivists'); identify with criminal culture; and become institutionalized in the sense that they function best within the highly controlled world of prison. Furthermore, imprisonment carries a substantial stigma in British society, and ex-offenders have great difficulty getting jobs and loans, making it more likely that they will resort again to crime.

Another aim of imprisonment, which is usually more implicit than explicit, is that prisons are there less to deter regular offenders from crime and more to control ordinary members of society. Foucault believed that far from being marginal institutions prisons are at the centre of our society and have developed systems of control that are taken up by other institutions – like schools and hospitals.[7] An anonymous ex-Home Office researcher made this point powerfully, and in language less difficult than that of Foucault, in the programme to David Hare's play 'Murmuring Judges', an analysis of Britain's criminal justice system:[8]

> So what do we conclude about the criminal justice system? Prison certainly doesn't work: seventy or eighty percent of prisoners will reoffend within the next two years. Prison encourages violent crime, it's a university of violence. If you can decrease the prison population, you will decrease crime. It's hugely expensive. So what is the function of criminal justice? It has a dramatist's function. It exists to say: we disapprove. It has a rhetorical power. Prison cannot be practical, so the criminal justice system is mainly symbolic. In the old

> days, the men in wigs marched through the town to the assizes. And that, basically, is what the apparatus of the law does now.

The most confused thinking of all surrounds the question of whether prison can reform and rehabilitate prisoners. We all very much want to believe that it can. The government which spends huge sums on prisons and the staff who spend their lives working in prisons would obviously like to believe that prisons have a positive side to them and that their time and money are being expended to a useful end. This must be particularly true of doctors and other health professionals working in prisons: they come from a sector where the sense of doing good is one of the major rewards. Yet most of the evidence shows that prisons cannot reform and rehabilitate.

The idea that prisons might be used positively can be traced back to Jeremy Bentham and Elizabeth Fry and entered British government thinking with the Gladstone Committee of 1895. The idea grew slowly, and in 1921 the Commissioners of Prisons wrote:

> The opinion has been growing in intensity for some years that mental and physical disabilities may largely contribute to the commission of crime.[9]

They wondered

> Whether some form of treatment rather than punishment by imprisonment can be devised which shall be more scientific, efficacious, and humane.

One upshot of this thinking was that in 1933 Dr W. H. de B. Hubert was appointed to try out psychological treatments at Wormwood Scrubs. He concluded, together with Dr Norbert East, in 1939:

> Psychotherapy as an adjunct to an ordinary prison sentence appears to be effective in preventing ... future antisocial behaviour.... The main object of psychotherapy in criminal work is to prevent crime being committed and repeated by the individual.[10]

The idea that prisons might be agents of reform had its heyday in the 1960s. The Home Office wrote in a White Paper of 1959, *Penal Practice in a Changing Society*: 'The constructive function of our prisons is to prevent the largest number of those committed to their care from offending again.'[11] This was to be achieved 'through more precise methods of classification and continual search for improved techniques ... and by more personal training'. Psychiatry was to be available in all prisons, and a psychiatric prison was to be built. 'The value of psychiatry is not limited to the treatment of those abnormal states of mind which require the kind of psychotherapy that will be given in the new establishment. A psychiatrically experienced doctor can do much to help disturbed prisoners not only to adjust themselves to prison life but also to change their general attitudes so that they make a better adjustment to society after release.' In 1969 the Court of Appeal ruled that 'It may be perfectly proper to increase the sentence to enable a cure for alcoholism to be undertaken whilst in prison.'

The idea that crime should be treated in some psychiatric manner has always been particularly strong in the case of women. Our culture is deeply threatened by female crime as it clashes so strongly with the stereotypes of women as mothers and carers, and the tendency has thus been to see criminal women as sick and in need of treatment. A Home Office report released in 1970 said: 'It may well be that as the end of the century draws nearer penological process will result in even fewer women or no women at all being given prison sentences.'[12] New plans were produced in 1971 for Holloway, the major women's prison, and it was to be built like a hospital; and a woman doctor, Lady Megan Bull, was encouraged to become governor in 1971 even though she had only very limited experience of prisons.

There have always, however, been doubts about the ability of prisons to reform and rehabilitate, particularly among those working full-time in the prisons. Sir Godfrey Lushington, permanent secretary at the Home Office at the time of the Gladstone Committee, said prison cannot reform because of 'the crushing of self respect ... the continued association with none but criminals ... and the denial of liberty'.[13] This view has prevailed. Nobody has been able to demonstrate that prison can reform, and a mountain of empirical evidence shows that it cannot.[14]

The idea that prison is essentially bad has become mainstream, and Norval Morris, the American criminologist, has advocated as a result a policy called humane containment.[15] The policy has three basic aims: minimal use of custody; minimal use of security; and normalization of the prison. This policy has gained widespread acceptance, but the government-appointed May Committee of 1979 was strongly against it: 'Humane containment', it said, "has the fatal defect of being a means without an end. Prisons would become human warehouses for both inmates and staff, leaving prison staff in a moral vacuum where routine brutalisation would become the order of the day.'[16] It concluded: 'The rhetoric of "treatment and training" has had its day ... but the rhetoric alone should be changed and not all the admirable and constructive things that are done in its name.'

The May Committee wanted rule 1 of the prison service rewritten. It read – and still reads – 'The purpose of the training and treatment of convicted prisoners shall be to encourage and assist them to lead a good and useful life.' The committee wanted it to read: 'The purpose of the detention of convicted prisoners shall be to keep them in custody which is both secure and yet positive, and to that end the behaviour of all the responsible authorities shall be such as to: a) Create an environment which can assist them to respond and contribute to society as positively as possible; b) preserve and promote their self respect; c) minimise, to the degree of security necessary in each particular case, the harmful effects of their removal from normal life; d) prepare them for and assist them on discharge.'[16]

The Woolf Report of 1991, which was a response to the prison riots of 1990 and has been greeted as the most radical report on prisons for decades, looked favourably on this statement and on the Prison Department's statement of purpose, but wanted more emphasis on prisons as part of the criminal justice system, justice for prisoners, and prisoners taking responsibility for their actions.[2] But it said: 'We are not suggesting ... a return to what came to be known as the treatment model of imprisonment ... while we would not suggest that an offender should be sentenced to imprisonment for reformative treatment, we regard it as part of the Prison Service's role to ensure ... that a prisoner ... should have an opportunity of training.'

We can conclude that prison will keep dangerous people out of the way but at a substantial price; does not deter offenders but may have some controlling effect on society at large; does provide punishment, but the punishment consists of more than the simple taking away of liberty; and does not reform and rehabilitate, although it is hard for those associated with prisons to drop the idea altogether.

When the purpose of imprisonment is so unclear, it is only to be expected that the purpose of the prison medical services will also be unclear. And the lack of clarity impedes development in the services and makes it hard for them to relate to the broader medical world and recruit high-quality health professionals into the service – particularly when there is real doubt over just what influence the medical services have within the broader service and how much the health professionals are serving the prison authorities rather than the patients.

The idea that the job of prison medical services is to treat prisoners and make them less likely to offend is, at least for now, dead, but this was the view of Dr Ian Pickering, who was Director of the Prison Medical Service until 1976. He wanted to recruit doctors with psychiatric experience. His successor, Dr Jim Orr, in contrast thought that the service should concentrate on supplying general practitioner services to prisoners.

But even when the idea of treating prisoners to reduce their chances of re-offending is dead, some doctors still believe that a primary function of the services should be to provide psychological treatments to those many prisoners with psychological problems. Some of these doctors, particularly those working in special units like that at Barlinnie Prison or the Wormwood Scrubs Annexe for sex offenders and prisoners with drug problems, would even accept the suggestion that such treatment might reduce the chances of somebody re-offending – although this would be a 'side-effect' of the treatment. Other doctors are reluctant to provide any sort of psychological treatment to prisoners for fear of seeming to condone the idea of mentally disordered people being kept in prison.

Providing reactive general practitioner services has usually been a function of prison medical services, but often these have been supplied by general practitioners who work primarily in the outside community. This may be particularly important if normalization is to be an objective of the prison service, and the debate is continuing on how much such services should be supplied by prison doctors and how much by outside doctors.

Despite the captive population and the high prevalence of health problems among prisoners, prison medical services have had little tradition of supplying preventative services. This is probably partly because of anxieties that prisoners might see this somehow as an invasion by 'prison authorities' and more, I suspect, because the slow-changing medical services in prison have been slow to follow the well-established trend in the medical services in the community to shift more towards prevention. Again, preventive services might best be provided by those working mainly outside the prisons.

There has also been debate over how much prisons should provide specialist medical services. Traditionally, they have provided dental, optical, pharmacy, and radiological services within many prisons and surgical, genito-urinary, and obstetric services within some prisons. Often these services have been provided because it has been administratively easier to provide them within the prisons. But doubts about the quality of some of these services and about whether or not the medical services should be providing them have led to reappraisal. There have also been discussions about concentrating prisoners with particular conditions – for instance, diabetes – in particular prisons staffed with doctors with specialist experience in that condition. But would it make sense to send prisoners to a particular prison simply because they are diabetic? And how would this fit with treating prisoners more humanely in local prisons?

A function of the prison medical services that has consumed much of their time has been to prepare reports for courts and the parole board. But increasingly these reports are being provided outside prison, avoiding expensive and destructive imprisonment. And the role of providing such reports conflicts with the caring role. How can a prisoner consult a doctor about a tricky problem in the morning, knowing that the information might be relevant to a parole board report that the same doctor will be preparing in the afternoon?

These conflicts become even more severe when we consider the role of doctors in the punishment of prisoners. For doctors to declare prisoners 'fit for punishment' is clearly a conflict of interest, and in the mind of prisoners the doctors examining prisoners in punishment cells and declaring them unharmed is more a semantic than a real difference. Prisoners do generally regard prison doctors as having a greater allegiance to the prison authorities than the prisoners. They are 'them' not 'us' in a world starkly divided between them and us. This differentiation has been even more acute in times when prison doctors have been obliged to force-feed hunger-striking prisoners.

Providing environmental and public health services has been a function of the prison medical services – despite few of the prison doctors having any special training. This function can also create conflict of interest as doctors are then seen to be condoning squalid conditions. These duties merge into doctors having managerial responsibilities within the prison system. Particularly when the idea that prisons could reform and rehabilitate has been in the ascendancy doctors have been closely involved in management. But often prison doctors have not had the necessary skills and there has been conflict with more strictly medical responsibilities.

The latest development in thinking about the function of prison medical services is that they should, in the jargon of the new NHS, become purchasers – with no responsibility for providing services but simply for purchasing them from the National Health Service or elsewhere. The oddly named Home Office Efficiency Scrutiny of 1990 called for the replacement of the prison medical service by a prison health service that would be a purchaser rather than a provider of health services.[17] A 'health director' would concentrate on advice, policy formulation, strategic planning, setting and monitoring standards, promoting health care, training, and external representation. The director would be supported by area physicians and clinical managers. The Scrutiny thought that these changes would end the isolation of prison medicine, increase reassurance to the public, match need and provision, and create a clear distinction between clinical and management roles. These proposals were accepted by the Home Office but have been implemented only in part. The renamed Health Service for Prisoners is still providing services not just purchasing them.

I have argued elsewhere that the Home Office should consider not only implementing the full Scrutiny proposals but also going further and handing over purchasing to the NHS.[18] This could have real advantages. First, combinations of district health authorities and family health service authorities are busy developing purchasing skills in a way that the prison medical service will be hard put to match. Second, the purchasers have access to the public health skills that have been lacking in prisons. Third, the purchasing authorities should be able to purchase for prisoners at the same time as purchasing for the rest of the community and so get a broader range of services at better prices. Fourth, the separation between the custodial and caring function would then be complete and the recurrent conflicts of interest would be abolished.

The confusions over the purpose of imprisonment and the purpose and function of prison medical services generates confusion in how health problems are tackled in prison. I want now to explore some examples.

Suicide is a longstanding and currently increasing problem in British prisons. Public and political concern has led to several reports on this issue.[19,20] One response is that prison is an environment where every aspect of the prisoner's life is controlled and that prisons and prison doctors must stop people killing themselves by placing them in strip cells if necessary. But another view is that the principles of justice and responsibility mean that rather than controlling prisoners more you aim to create conditions where people are unlikely to kill themselves. In other words, you encourage cultural change. Where should prison doctors stand in this debate and what is their power to implement what they decide? In fact, the voice of prison doctors has been hardly heard in the debate.

The response of prisons to HIV infection has often been poor. Within the punitive and highly judgemental culture of prisons both staff and inmates have tended to isolate, blame and victimize those infected with HIV. Prison doctors with their low status and confused mission have often been powerless to prevent these wrongheaded policies. Similarly doctors have not been able to insist on the distribution of condoms within prisons. The authorities have adopted the legalistic and restricted view that to distribute condoms would be to condone intercourse between men, which is illegal in prisons although legal in the outside world. Again doctors have been powerless and confused.

A longer-standing problem is over treating sex offenders and drug and alcohol abusers in prison. Many prisoners have such problems, but treatment facilities within prisons are often poor or non-existent. One problem of current prison doctors – poised uncomfortably and confusingly between prisoners and prison authorities – is over the quality of consent for whatever treatment is available. Do prisoners consent to such treatment because they want it or because they think that they will lose privileges – like parole – if they don't? Another problem is that treating sex offenders in an environment devoid of women and drug and alcohol abusers in a prison (at least theoretically) without both substances is peculiar and unlikely to produce long-term success. Should therefore prison doctors be fighting for more normal conditions in order to make treatment more real? Or should they insist that treatment takes place outside prisons?

A problem that creates a continuing headache for prison authorities and doctors is the management of mothers and babies in prison. Prison is a poor environment for young children, and it's also an environment in which mothers find it difficult to develop their mothering skills because dependence rather than independence is the norm. Should doctors demand, as the *British Medical Journal* has done,[21] that everything possible is done to release women with babies and small children? Or is such a policy unjust to women without babies? Should doctors at least demand that mothers with babies be given access to better conditions and more responsibility than other prisoners? Or should they at least avoid encouraging the dependence habitual in prisons but which is harmful to motherhood?

A further conflict arises for doctors over the related issues of research and audit. It is almost axiomatic in medicine that research and audit are necessary to raise understanding and standards. Yet research and audit are rare in prisons, and when they do happen it is usually under the aegis of outside academics. Again prison doctors worry about the quality of informed consent for any research, but this often sounds like an excuse rather than a real reason for not conducting research. Research and audit may be inimical to the culture of prison authorities, but they are essential for high-quality health care.

These problems – and many more like them – confront prison medical services all the time. I believe that they will never be adequately addressed while the purpose of imprisonment remains unclear, the job of the health service for prisoners is also unclear, and the relationship of doctors to prison authorities is ambiguous. What we need is broad debate on the purposes of imprisonment and a health service for prisoners provided by doctors and other health professionals who are ultimately employed by the NHS rather than the Home Office. If those working in the Health Service for Prisoners were responsible to the NHS they could then clarify their own mission even if the mission of the prisons themselves remains cloudy.

Notes

1. Smith, R., *Prison health care* (London: BMA, 1984).
2. Woolf, H. and Tumim, S., *Prison disturbances April 1990* (London: HMSO, 1991). (Woolf Report).
3. House of Commons Social Services Committee, *Prison Medical Service* (London: HMSO, 1986).
4. Working Party of the Royal College of Physicians, *Report to the Chief Medical Officer, March 1989. The prison medical service in England and Wales: recruitment and training of doctors* (London: Home Office and Department of Health, 1990).
5. European Committee for the Prevention of Torture and Inhuman Degrading Treatment or Punishment, *Report to the United Kingdom Government on the visit to the United Kingdom* (Strasburg: Council of Europe, 1991).
6. Departmental Committee on Prisons, *Report* (London: HMSO, 1895) (Cmnd 7702). (Gladstone Report).
7. Foucault, M., *Discipline and Punish* (London: Allen Lane, 1977).
8. Anonymous, Programme to *Murmuring Judges* by David Hare (London: National Theatre, 1992).
9. Commissioners of Prisons, *Report 1919–20* (London: HMSO, 1921).
10. East, W. N. and Hubert, W. H. de B., *The Psychological Treatment of Crime* (London: HMSO, 1939).
11. Home Office, *Penal Practice in a Changing Society* (London: HMSO, 1959).
12. Home Office, *Treatment of Women and Girls in Custody* (London: HMSO, 1970).
13. Departmental Committee on Prisons, *Report* (London: HMSO, 1895).
14. Brody, S. R., *The Effectiveness of Sentencing*, Home Office Research Study no. 35 (London: HMSO, 1976).
15. Morris, N., *The Future of Imprisonment* (Chicago: University of Chicago Press, 1974).
16. Committee of Inquiry into the United Kingdom Prison Services, *Report* (London: HMSO, 1979).

17. Smith, R., 'Arise the new prison service', *BMJ* (1990) 301: 892–3. Lygo R.
18. Smith, R., 'Prison medicine: beginning again', *BMJ* (1992) 304: 134–5.
19. Her Majesty's Chief Inspector of Prisons for England and Wales, *Suicide and Self Harm in Prison Establishments in England and Wales* (London: HMSO, 1990).
20. Lloyd, C., *Suicide and Self Injury in Prison: A Literature Review* (London: HMSO, 1990); see, also, the chapter by Liebling and Ward, in this volume.
21. Dillner, S., Keeping Babies in Prison, *BMJ* (1992).304: 932–33.

Commentary

Smith It occurred to me that there is probably no better way in Britain to have a sense of going back in time than to go into a prison. They seem like extraordinarily ancient institutions – which I think is due partly to the smell, partly the squalor, partly the fact that a lot of them were built in the middle of the last century: and more than anything else, it is the kind of attitudes that you come across there. And I then had a picture (which comes from one of the reports of the Chief Inspector of Prisons): it is of a prisoner standing before a doctor. The prison doctor still has his overcoat on. He does not look up at the prisoner and there is a warder (I should not call him that but somehow I always do) who stands beside the doctor. The prisoner calls the doctor Sir, and the doctor calls him by his surname.

Dr John Sinclair I am a prison medical officer and I think I can speak for the great majority of us and say that we are highly committed, desperately committed, to producing a better health service for prisons, and we believe that we really are at a watershed now. The time has come for us to get out of the Prison Service and into the National Health Service or perhaps into a special health authority in the Department of Health. My question is addressed to you, Judge: Do you see managerial problems if doctors work for the National Health Service in the future?

Tumim I see managerial problems if you do not have the equivalent of hospital managers deployed in relation to prisons. I think one of the difficulties of the prison health care service is a lack of management. There have been no doubt admirable doctors and diagnoses and so on, not management: that is one reason why you have these extraordinarily unpopular hospitals in some prisons: nasty and squalid. Whether you operate through a buying-in system, which is the fashionable way of going to the National Health Service, or not does not seem to me to make much difference. I'm looking purely pragmatically at the difficulty of turning the prison medical service into a part of the National Health Service, the difficulty on which Sir Donald Acheson was advising the Health Care Service. I think what you want to do is to get some better management, the provision of hospital managers, to look at the estate problems and so on, and rationalizing the beds to provide accommodation where you need it, with the specialists available. I do not really care whether you spend your money 'buying in' or whether it is done through managers brought in to the Health Service.

Tumim (In response to a question) I think there is a great difficulty for the prison governor in trying to run an institution with a lot of professional people responsible to their professional bosses rather than to him. When you have some problem about the hospital the governor says I dare not interfere otherwise my civil servant will say it is a matter for higher medical authority and not for me. I would support moves to give the prison governor more authority and certainly a bigger budget. I think it is astonishing that a head master of a school can splash paint all over the place while the governor of a prison cannot. This seems to me to be unfortunate. I can see the difficulty where he has to turn to different people for different purposes. Clearly if it's a question of whether it is appropriate to use a certain drug, that has to be decided by the medical officer within the medical context. But there are quite a lot of other problems which are borderline: the state of hygiene for example. When you go to the splendid new establishment at Woolwich you find a very high percentage of cells in the hospital block which have no lavatory accommodation or sanitation and will not get any: you find hooks which look as though designed for suicide: you find there has been a bad design system and the medical staff were not brought in. This is a problem where you have different lines of credibility, different lines of accountability.

Michael Farrar I am involved in Yorkshire in linking our purchases in the NHS with the purchases in the prisons, and I think that is going to contribute significantly. But one thing does concern me in some of the prisons that I am aware of, where prisoners have access to a shower once a week and have access to a change of underwear at longer intervals, and if you want to improve the health status of prisoners then perhaps you should not necessarily look at health care provision, you should look at the environmental health conditions within that prison. You could do far more in terms of creating a culture of dignity within the prison, which in some ways might ultimately lead to the development by prisoners themselves of some greater self-respect, which in my view is probably the key determinant in health status, not necessarily the kind of health care which is received.

Smith Of course you are absolutely right. That is also true in the community, where provision of health care has little impact on health, which is affected by all sorts of social conditions.

Speaker My experience as a consultant in the Health Service is that the management is hardly one of outstanding success. They may block contracts that expire in November or December and leave hospitals with unutilized facilities. I do not think they have got it right at all. I suspect that the person who has to purchase the health care, from whatever the source, should be the governor.

Smith I do not see how the governor could know what health care is needed. But with resources which are limited, I think that the notion of purchasing – being able to sit down and think about what it is we want to purchase among various competing schemes – has attractions. Do we want to purchase a smoking prevention programme or do we want to purchase more coronary by-pass surgery?

Sim I would just like to say that I can't really settle on the argument that we should purchase health care. I think that a purchasing agreement is anathema to the spirit of the 1946 Act. And it has led to all sorts of problems – one of which was indicated in the *Guardian* the other day about a patient who died an undignified death in the out-patient department after seven hours on a trolley. What it means is that those people or those groups that have been marginal like prisoners will become even more marginal. People get hung up on purchasing – shall we purchase this or purchase that - –and neglect the fundamental issues. For example, no one has mentioned the issue of training for medical orderlies in prisons which is less than satisfactory - and these are the persons who come face to face with prisoners. This is fundamental to delivery of health care and their training is, shall we say, problematic.

Smith How can you argue for what we have had for the last 40 years – it has got us nowhere. It is because of that system that it is acceptable to have people working in prisons with such poor, impoverished training. The problems that you are attaching to purchasing – and I am not speaking out strongly in favour – are due to underfunding. There is at least the potential with the concept of on the purchasing to consider our priorities. It seems ludicrous to have these people who are so poorly trained, and it would be incumbent purchasers to consider their training and the training of the medical officers who are employed to provide the health care.

Speaker The only conversation I have ever heard about purchasing services from outside agencies between a manager of a prison hospital and somebody else was: 'Can we afford another member of staff or do we increase the amount of medication used to control the prisoners'. That was a question of budget, and we are talking about a prison environment where a certain minimal amount of control is required, and has to be provided in certain circumstances by the medical services; and if it comes down to an issue of priority, staff or medication, I think we have a potentially very serious problem on our hands.

Smith It is a grossly simplified argument to suggest that the practice stems from separating purchasing from providing. I think a lot of problems flow from lack of resources. Surely you are not arguing for the kind of monolithic system we have had in previous years. What is the alternative?

Sim The Act of 1946 with its problems and the various faults in the system did at least institute some kind of nationalized health care. People talk to me about agencies. My argument to that is that the National Health Service has never been tried as it should have been tried: rehabilitation for instance has never been put into practice in the way that it should: and what we are likely to get in the future is the Americanization of the system to the detriment of some very positive things.

Speaker There is an analogous situation in the provision of medical services to the armed forces. I am old enough to have done National Service back in 1956. In the last 20 or 30 years the Service hospitals have been closing down and the civilian medical practitioners have been brought in. The medical service to the armed forces (in peace) has become civilianized in a way that you seem to be wanting for the prison service.

Speaker Within the last 30 years civilian consultants have been appointed to the medical services of the armed forces and the tendency has been to transfer service patients to a civilian hospital for specialized treatment.

Dr Michael Whitelaw To what extent has scandal and exposure been responsible for reform, rather than enlightenment or scientific methods? I was interested in Dr Sim's comment about the pressures on many of the people to prevent them from speaking out. And of course Richard Smith has written a leader in the *BMJ* about what happens to whistle-blowers. It seems to me that the combination of the Official Secrets Act, and what happens to whistle-blowers, would prevent informed professionals within the system speaking out about the abuses that they know of, and therefore shaping some proper policy; and unless we embrace that, and have a Freedom of Information Act, we will go on with reflex responses, and Kenneth Clarke announcing things which clearly this room realizes are nonsense.

Shaw I think a very important point made by Judge Tumim is that it might be really helpful if medical officers working in prisons were willing to speak out publicly about some of these issues. And one of the factors behind the campaign to make prison medical care part of the National Health Service has been the thought that doctors whose career structure was within the National Health Service might be more willing to do that.

9

The Criminal Lunatic Asylum System Before and After Broadmoor

Sir Louis Blom-Cooper, QC

The tri-correlates of the bad, the mad and the high-security closed institution, as they became expressed in the shape and form of the criminal lunatic asylum system of the second half of the nineteenth century, have been the dominating theme of our society's approach to the confinement of mentally disordered offenders. I suppose in Butlerian terms, one might say, mentally abnormal offenders, or I think in the current jargon, difficult-to-manage patients. But I think I am going to stick to mentally disordered offenders. I have grown up with that rubric.

Abandonment of that system, not yet complete, is, I think, of very recent origin. The type of prisoners compulsorily detained has always varied, reflecting medico-legal concepts of insanity, mental illness and mental handicap again, in contemporary language, persons with learning disabilities, but I shall stick to mental handicap as being more familiar to me. They were all accompanied by social attitudes to dangerous conduct. Dangerousness, pithily described by Dr Peter Scott, is a very dangerous concept. Dangerousness was, initially at any rate, linked ineluctably with insanity, at least when manifested in the commission of serious crime, mostly homicide, which justified incarceration of the offender beyond that required for the general run of psychiatrically-ill patients in the county asylums. Great public understanding of dangerousness in mentally disordered offenders has emerged with the development of the forensic psychiatric services of recent years.

Historically, though, the appropriate legal framework for mentally disordered offenders and disruptive psychiatric patients within civil categories has depended upon whether this position is conceived in essentially penal or therapeutic terms. This was never more so in the provision of the institution. The forms of security employed to contain the perceived dangers of mentally disordered offenders have not changed dramatically over the last century: perimeter security in the shape of high, forbidding walls, internal locks and bars, individual control and restraint, by both physical and mechanical means, and removal of association from fellow inmates by the use of seclusion. They have all been there over the whole of the century. All of these features of the criminal lunatic asylum have, to a greater or lesser extent, been in continuous use in various guises up to the present day.

The ethos of Broadmoor, the first criminal lunatic asylum, built in England in 1863 and I remind those who come from across the water, was a copy of the successful establishment of Dundrum which was built in 1852 by the Irish. The first criminal lunatic asylum in England, Broadmoor, still pervades the practices adopted in the Special Hospitals which statutorily, organizationally, and managerially are part of our mental health system. It is little wonder that Special Hospitals are regarded by the public as prison hospitals, since they are so-described so often by some ill-informed members of our judiciary. How is it that modern attitudes to the care and treatment of the mentally disordered have not managed to discard outdated and outmoded practices, redolent of the institutions for the criminal lunatic?

The common law of England, as early as 1482, had established that it was lawful to incarcerate a dangerous lunatic, either in his own home or in the local bridewell. It was much later, in the Vagrancy Act of 1714, that Parliament provided for two Justices of the Peace to direct persons described as, and I am quoting, 'furiously mad and dangerous to be kept safely locked up and if the Justices found it necessary, to be there chained'. A later Vagrancy Act of 1744 spoke of 'curing such persons during such restraint'. The implicit focus of eighteenth-century legislation was that magistrates were capable of identifying the dangerous insane and of deciding when they could be safely discharged. There was no medical intervention in the process of incarceration, indeed none was envisaged.

By the late eighteenth century the process of lunacy reform had become an issue to which a considerable degree of governmental attention was devoted. Its main aims were: 1) to prevent abuse and ill-treatment of the insane; 2) to ensure proper care, preferably in special institutions; and 3) to prevent sane persons from being defamed as lunatics. Consequently, from the early part of the nineteenth century, this process of confining the insane gradually diminished to the present level of less than 5 per cent of the mentally disordered in hospitals. As is often the case, sensational happenings, involving individual and often unsuspecting players, can often turn into the catalysts that lead to fundamental changes in a society's perception or attitude to specific areas of social or health policy. Just such an event occurred on 15 May, 1800, when James Hatfield discharged a pistol at King George III, as he was entering the Royal Box at the Drury Lane Theatre. Subsequently, a jury found Hatfield 'not guilty, by reason of insanity' on a charge of high treason. Such a verdict was at that time unprecedented. Hatfield's acquittal was due in no small measure to the brilliance of his advocate, Thomas Erskine, later to become Lord Chancellor Erskine. He addressed the jury in these words, which I would like you to listen to for a moment, spoken not by Erskine, but a latterday humbler lawyer. He said:

> it is time indeed that in some, perhaps in many cases, the human mind is stormed in its citadel and laid prostrate under the stroke of frenzy. Those unhappy sufferers, however, are not so much considered by physicians as maniacs, as to be in a state of delirium from fever. There indeed all the ideas are overwhelmed. For reason is not merely disturbed, but driven wholly from her seat. But these cases are not only extremely rare, but can never become the subject of judicial difficulty. In other cases, reason is not driven from the seat, but distraction sits down upon it with her, holds her, trembling upon it, and frightens her from her propriety.

The meaning of this powerful passage is very important, not least because it distinguished between those whose minds were so disordered as to be totally deprived of memory and understanding, and those who, while retaining possession of their mental faculties, were nevertheless severely disabled, by what Erskine termed 'distraction'. The Attorney General, relying on the institutional authorities such as Coke and Hale, seventeenth-century legal luminaries, both judges, had argued that *dementia naturales* or idiocy alone could place a man in this helpless condition. Erskine, much ahead of his time I think, was advancing the now-familiar argument that offenders, however severe their mental disorder which afflicts them, have both reason and memory. Indeed, they form the large majority of mentally disordered offenders; the kind of asocial condition of incomprehension or delusion identified by the jurist was always a rare exception. If Erskine could come back for a brief look at crime today and the treatment of offenders, much, perhaps too much, would appear familiar to him. But he would gain a lot of satisfaction from his great forensic triumph. If the law in 1800 was essentially pre-scientific and quasi-medieval in its approach, the Criminal Lunatics Act of that year, reacting strongly and speedily to the Hatfield acquittal, marked the critical beginning of the law relating to the mentally disordered offender. Hatfield's case had followed the attempt, 12 years earlier, on the King's life, by a Margaret Nicholson. Parliament, in 1800, then hurriedly passed a law 'for the safe custody of insane persons charged with offences'. Courts were given the duty to detain such persons in custody, in those now famous words, 'During His/Her Majesty's Pleasure'.

The seemingly inevitable delays between recommendation and provision, endemic in dealing with mentally disordered offenders, ensued. Previous legislation assumed that lunatics would be confined, providing specific authority for the detention of dangerous and criminal lunatics, language used in the Acts of 1744 and 1800 respectively. The Parliamentary Select Committee of 1807, appointed to inquire into the state of the criminal and pauper lunatics in England reported that there were approximately 37 people in jails under the 1800 Act, predicting that this figure was likely to rise. The Committee felt that this was extremely unsatisfactory, negatively affecting not only the recovery of the insane, but also the security and comfort of the other prisoners.

It was against this backcloth that in 1810 the Bethlem Hospital in London was asked by the Home Office if it would set aside space to cater for a facility for 'criminal lunatics'. This criminal lunatic asylum facility, although funded by the Exchequer, remained in the control of the parent hospital. By October 1816 it was completed, providing 45 male and 15 female beds. This was expanded in 1837 at the government's request by 30 male beds. By 1838 these were filled. I like to call this term, and I shall come back to it again, as Crowthorne's disease, and some will realize that that's a reference to a mental health variant of Parkinson's law, when an institution expands proportionately to meet the extent of a perceived need. And perhaps that ought to be quoted to the present Home Secretary.

Many of the inmates of the Bethlem Hospital became the first occupants of the criminal lunatic asylum built at Broadmoor in 1863. Dr Helps, who was the resident physician at Bethlem described the transfer of the 112 patients 'without a single casualty'. He added, and I am grateful to our chairman, Dr Henry Rollin, for the quote from his most delightful little book *Festina Lente*: 'We are much indebted to the authorities of the South-Western Railway who successfully made every arrangement for their comfort and safe transfer from Bethlem down to Broadmoor.'

The most famous transferee was, of course, Daniel McNaughton, who had been charged with the murder of Sir Robert Peel's secretary and, like Hatfield, was acquitted on the grounds of insanity. But he's not alone in having achieved fame. The other famous name is Richard Dadd, who lived from 1817 to 1886, some 69 years, and was declared insane at the age of 26 when he was just beginning to make his name as one of the most talented artists of his generation. After killing his father in 1843, he spent the remaining 43 years of his life, first in Bethlem and then in Broadmoor, where he died. He continued to paint throughout his detention during Her Majesty's Pleasure and when he was 54 he painted a picture called *The Wayside Inn*. Its subject is a country inn, overlooking a small hill town with a distant plain beyond. In the foreground a mounted traveller discusses his route with the landlord of the inn. It was a rarity among Dadd's work from this period, in that it shows a scene from everyday life realistically portrayed, even by somebody who by then had been incarcerated some 13 years in Broadmoor and previously in Bethlem. The Bethlem Hospital archives are the principal centre for research on the life and work of Richard Dadd. Last year the National Heritage Memorial Fund assisted the purchase of this fascinating picture with a grant of £24,000. Had Dadd committed his crime 100 years later, we would surely not have had to spend some of the country's money purchasing a painting which would not have gone to other sources, a painting which, as I say, was done over half a normal life span in captivity.

The urge to establish a separate institution for the criminally insane had begun two decades earlier before 1863. The Metropolitan Commissioners in Lunacy in 1844 published the results of a two-year survey covering all licensed houses, public and private, in England and Wales. The Commissioners' survey revealed that there were approximately 342 criminal patients confined in asylums, jails and the, by then, enlarged Bethlem Hospital. They concluded that there could be special provisions for persons described as criminal lunatics. Their report was soon followed by the Lunatics Act of 1845. This was an important piece of reforming legislation, which among other things created the Commissioners in Lunacy. They were accountable to the Lord Chancellor and empowered to inspect and report on all licensed institutions that housed lunatics. The Act of 1845 was not especially forthcoming with regard to the management of criminal lunatics.

The Creation of Broadmoor

The Lunatics Act of 1860 provided the authority for the building of Broadmoor Criminal Lunatic Asylum at Crowthorne in Berkshire, some 30 miles from London. Building began in March 1863, utilizing prison labour, that is to say 250 prisoners and their officers were transferred from Portsmouth, Portland and Chatham and, amazingly, it was finished by the end of that year. From the outset Broadmoor encountered problems. After 12 months, the Commissioners felt that there was a need for more female beds. Dr Meyer, the first medical superintendent, transferred and rejected six female patients 'because of their troublesome and violent behaviour', and in 1867 the Commissioners in Lunacy were advised that future admissions would be restricted to HMP offenders, that is being held during Her Majesty's Pleasure, offenders who had become insane after conviction. No matter how dangerous they were, prisoners in county jails would have to be treated in county asylums. It was clear from the Commissioners' report at that time that they felt that this stance not only undermined the precise reasons for the creation of Broadmoor, but was also not consistent with the intention of the legislation.

A year later Dr Meyer was again at the thick end of the Commissioners' tongue. After their annual visit to Broadmoor on 14 October, 1868, the Commissioners wrote in their 23rd Report in language which was, for all its florid Victorian circumlocutions, a pungent attack on the practice of seclusion and I should like to quote from that:

> Of the violent and even dangerous propensities of some of the patients placed in these wards and of the generally unfavourable character of the rest, there is no doubt, but it is a matter of the gravest doubt whether insane persons of the criminal class having this disposition should be treated differently from other patients suffering under mental diseases. The experience of the Commissioners has led them to the conclusion that patients of the most refractory classes are amenable to the influences which, by general consent, are now employed in the treatment as well as the most acute as of the mildest forms of mental disorder, and that it is both expedient and safe to extend to them under vigilant and incessant supervision the same kind of advantage, if indeed the withholding of all indulgence were more likely that the concession of it to have a beneficial effect there's nothing in the class of cases in this asylum that should intercept on any ground of personal considerational sympathy an application of the repressive system to the fullest extent. But in other times there has been sufficient trial of that system on all descriptions of patients and in every conceivable state of circumstances and it has uniformly failed as completely as the other and succeeded in more or less degree. It has been found all but invariably that by association with others, by some occupation as far as practicable, by the prospect of time to time some recreation or amusement, above all by regular daily outdoor exercise,

> improvement has been made in the habits of the most inveterate and in the most evil dispositions. No attempts of this kind are now made at Broadmoor. If a patient exhibits violent conduct, he is for so many days, or portions of days, put into seclusion. He is supposed to be or has been given proof of being dangerous, he is isolated altogether. To none set apart as refractory are the arrangements applied which make judicious and satisfactory provision for the bulk of the inmates by suitable accommodation and considerable treatment. The accepted class occupy cheerless rooms, have neither occupation nor amusement, are subjected to the unrelieved and continued presence of gloomy and dispiriting influences, have no opportunity at any time of associating with patients in the other blocks, are confined for exercise to narrow airing courts within high walls and in some six or seven instances marked out for special example and even the class they form part are required to take such exercise alone.

I think we found something not very different at Ashworth in 1991. I end this quote with another part of what the Commissioners said because it shows the vigour of their language and that nothing very much has changed. They went on and said that 'this is not in our opinion an efficient way of dealing with the mental disease, however complicated with criminal habits and even dangerous violence we can see that our duty once more to put on record. But the same remonstrance in fact, having been made, unavailingly on every visit of the Commissioner since Broadmoor opened, and this is now 23 years on, it is with no expectation of any kind of present result that we repeat it now.'

My next title for this part of the address is Plus ça change. If the Commissioners had no expectation from Dr Meyer and his successors that the practice would be abandoned, the formers' inheritor, the Mental Health Act Commission, is now pursuing the recommendation of the Ashworth Hospital Inquiry report, that seclusion could, to employ the ringing words of Dr John Conolly in his great treatise of 1856 on the treatment of the insane without medical restraints,'be ended not only with safety but with incalculable advantage'.

From the outset Broadmoor was managed by the Home Office, which also controlled admissions and discharges. This historical connection with the Home Office and their role has frequently caused some degree of confusion to both members of the public and the professions involved in the care and treatment of this group of people. Special hospitals are not prison hospitals. All the patients are detained under mental health legislation, and indeed only two-thirds of whom are committed by the criminal courts, something people don't often realize. With rare exceptions Broadmoor Hospital never admitted patients described as mentally handicapped, and it was not until the Mental Health Act of 1959 that non-offender patients were admitted via the civil process of detention.

By 1892 it was reported that Broadmoor was full, and throughout the last decade of the nineteenth century it continued to operate to full capacity. Crowthorne's disease was about to break out again. It is ironic that it was the Lunacy Commissioners' Report of 1899 that raised the question 'of further accommodation for the criminal lunatics of the country, being of pressing importance'. The suggestion that another asylum should be built in the north of England appears to us to have some special advantage. Park Lane, now the northern part of Ashworth Hospital, was not built until the 1970s. The Commissioners had to wait three-quarters of a century. Broadmoor suffered yet another outbreak of Crowthorne's disease in 1900, by commencing construction of another block for 80 male patients. By 1903 the Lunacy Commissioners reported that Broadmoor was near to capacity. Despite providing accommodation for 566 men and 192 women, there were still 109 criminal lunatics in country asylums and 40 in HMP Parkhurst, all awaiting transfer to Broadmoor.

Due to the continuing concerns about these sorts of issues and the growing number of criminal lunatics waiting for transfer to Broadmoor criminal lunatic asylum, another asylum eventually emerged in 1912 at Rampton. It opened on 1 October, 1912, sited some 15 miles west of Lincoln in the remote Nottinghamshire countryside. It was described as a criminal lunatic asylum and managed by the Home Office. As with Broadmoor, it remained a criminal lunatic asylum until 1920 when its management control was passed to the Board of Control under the terms of the Mental Deficiency Act of 1913. This legislation served to provide for the supervision, protection and control of all mental defectives. Although the first transfers were from Broadmoor, these changes in provision influenced Rampton's development as a hospital for the mentally handicapped. Consequently, the new criminal lunatic asylum of the north soon became the first-stage institution for mental defectives with dangerous, violent and criminal propensities. The regime for this class of the mentally disordered offender was identical to that for the severely mentally ill.

By the early 1930s Rampton Hospital had suffered the effects of its own strain of Crowthorne's disease, that is to say, it had expanded over a period of time, to the point of being overcrowded. This situation was alleviated by the Board of Control repossessing Moss Side near Liverpool, intending to create a further state institution for mental defectives. In all, 101 men and women were then transferred from

Rampton to Moss Side. After the Second World War, in 1948, the ownership of Rampton and Moss Side was transferred to the Ministry of Health under Section 49 (4) of the National Health Service Act of 1946. Despite this change they continued to be managed by the Board of Control. Broadmoor was added to Rampton and Moss Side and the Ministry of Health. Unlike Rampton and Moss Side the criteria for admission and discharge of patients remained with the Home Office. The twin ministerial responsibilities have produced a continuing conflict of interests, one medically orientated, at least ostensibly, and the other, devoted to public protection.

Under Section 97 of the Mental Health Act of 1959, later repealed and replaced by Section 4 of the National Health Act of 1977, Broadmoor, Rampton and Moss Side became special hospitals, acquired to provide, as Dr McCullough, the last Medical Director of Park Lane described, for patients subject to detention who require treatment under conditions of special security on account of their dangerous, violent and criminal propensities. For the first time, the Special Hospitals came under the direct control of one organization, namely the Secretary of State for Health, at that time the Minister for the Department of Health and Social Security. The creation of a government agency in the shape of the Special Hospital Service Authority only came in October 1989.

By the middle of the twentieth century the Percy Commission reported, which led to the creation of the Mental Health Act of 1959. This replaced the vast amount of nineteenth-century legislation relating to criminal lunacy and mental deficiency. The 1959 Act brought revolutionary changes. Amongst those were: it allowed the majority of mentally disordered offenders to be admitted informally; it abolished most of the statutory distinctions between mental illness and deficiency; it obliged the Minister of Health to provide special hospitals, and it dissolved the old Board of Control. There was no supervisory or watchdog body until the Mental Health Act Commission came into existence in 1983.

Anticipating that there would be a difference in the volume and type of patients admitted to the Special Hospitals, Mr Enoch Powell, a very distinguished Minister of Health, created a working party to consider the role of the special hospitals and their interaction within the framework of the new mental health legislation and the mainstream National Health Service. Reporting in 1961 the Working Party stated that consideration should be given to further secure provision. They recommended that regional hospital boards be set up as a mixed economy of secure provision. The special needs of the mentally disordered offender were further focused on by the Butler Committee on Mentally Abnormal Offenders in 1975. Butler recommended the creation of 2,000 secure hospital beds below the level of security offered by the Special Hospitals. Parallel to this, the Glancy report of the year before proposed the creation of 1,000 secure provision beds. Those two reports led to the rise of the regional secure facilities, though over the last decade and a half they have provided less than half of the 2,000 places recommended by Butler. Today there are approximately only 650 beds in the RSUs and of course the Special Hospitals continue to contain large numbers of people who could be easily, readily housed in the regional secure units, Special Hospitals now housing something like 1,700 patients, of whom probably at least 60 per cent do not need the level of security which is provided.

A further result of the Butler Report was to recommend the creation of a fourth Special Hospital – Crowthorne's disease at work again, to help and relieve overcrowding in both the three existing Special Hospitals and prisons. In August 1979 Park Lane opened on a site adjacent to Moss Side in Liverpool. Complaints of abuse and maltreatment of patients were constant features of the Special Hospitals. Rampton Hospital was the subject of a major inquiry – that was the Boynton Report in 1980 – after the Yorkshire Television programme had exposed a number of major examples of bad professional practice. A number of nursing staff underwent criminal prosecution, all of them resulting in acquittals or convictions quashed by appellate courts. None of them at the end of the day was convicted.

Allegations of maltreatment continued to be raised throughout the 1980s and yet again a television programme, this time in March 1991, led to the Ashworth Inquiry. The Inquiry revealed (and I am quoting) 'a number of cases of improper nursing care and inadequate psychiatric service and failure on the part of management either to encourage, support or investigate the allegations properly'. The Inquiry went on: 'Our wider inquiry has revealed the hospital environment and culture which has given rise to numerous incidents, arising from an uncaring and demeaning attitude towards patients.' Employers have a duty to care for persons in their charge – 'a duty which has not been properly discharged', and the Inquiry ended up by describing Ashworth as 'a brutalising, stagnant, closed institution'.

The Ashworth Inquiry highlighted how strongly a large number of nursing staff associated themselves with the aims and values of the Prison Officers Association, of course, spilling over from the prison system. These values were rooted in an outdated philosophy of repressive and custodial care, rather than a genuine desire to deliver comprehensive, user-involved and sensitive service for the treatment of, and I use the phrase now, 'difficult-to-manage' patients suffering from mental disorders.

The High Security Working Group recently set up by the Secretary of State, under the chairmanship of Dr John Reed, is presently considering the future provision of care for this group of patients. There is a likelihood that in future mentally disordered offender patients may be offered care under a different model – that is to say, care and treatment should be as near as possible to the patient's home and family, and should follow the principle of employing the least restrictive alternative. To be able to achieve these objectives, it seems likely that not only may the number of referrals to Special Hospitals be reduced, and substantially reduced, but if the Reed Committee were to consider the creation of a number of units, and small ones, that is to say, for every two regional health authorities, it would be questionable whether there would be a need for three large Special Hospitals as we enter the twenty-first century.

My Conclusion

We stand at a watershed of the system for the care and treatment of mentally disordered offenders. To be able to move forward creatively, we need to learn from the mistakes of the past. Developing an effective service doesn't just mean more resources, a new model of delivering care, new buildings, new policies, etc. All these cannot replace a genuine awareness of the individual's needs and citizenship rights. Raising the civil status of detained patients would lessen the chances of their being treated inappropriately, with excessive restriction. As with prisoners in the penal system, so also detained patients do not lose their legal rights when they go into these institutions, save to the extent that any legislation takes them away.

To date, service planning has been disproportionately influenced by dependence on creating or expanding more institutional secure facilities, shaped by the historical belief that custodial care always provides the only solution to the problems of caring for the mentally disordered offender. The criminal lunatic asylum lives on in what I think is an attenuated, relabelled form. The Reed Committee needs to challenge this pattern of planning and spending. If not, I feel, sad to say, we may well have missed a great opportunity. We need to consider more new approaches, rather than indulge in tinkering with, or rehashing old ones. In facing the need for change, we are too often trapped by our history. The criminal lunatic asylum should be consigned to the museum of mental health. A fresh start should be made, establishing alternative models of a few, small high-security units in place of the existing, geographically isolated sites of the Special Hospitals.

10

The Woolf Report and After

Judge Stephen Tumim

In the *Woolf Report* of 1991 we said remarkably little about prison medical services, partly because we felt that such services were only very loosely connected with the disturbances of April 1990, and partly because a *Scrutiny Report on the Prison Medical Service* was then awaited. But we did state firmly: 'Prisoners and their families must feel confident that the medical treatment prisoners receive in prison is of comparable standard to that which they would receive in normal life from the National Health Service.' In one respect such treatment is often superior to what inmates would receive outside: access to medicine in prison is often far more prompt than in a hard-pressed community health centre. It is the quality of some of the treatment with which we must be concerned.

In 1992 there was an alteration in the arrangements for medical services which Joe Pilling, then Director-General, claimed as 'a celebration of change'. In my Annual Report for the year, I wrote as follows:

> The replacement of a Medical Service by a Health Care Service gives a far higher prominence to preventive medicine. It greatly extends the work of the Service. The Director has pledged it to more consultation of patients as to how they want things done. We must now expect, and indeed hope for, useful pronouncements and advice from the new Service in such areas as food and diet and hours of meals, the state of the kitchens, time out of cell, and the need for physical and mental exercise. The continuing lack of a gym for nearly a thousand remands at Brixton (the present gym being outside the secure area) is now a matter for health care comment by those working under the Director of Health Care. (Preface to *Annual Report 1991–1992*)

That change of attitude, proudly claimed, if it is to be a reality rather than a modish choice of language, leads me to try and look again at the standing of the prison doctor in relation to the Prison Service. We must note that the Health Care Service, the old Prison Medical Service, has an astonishing number of admirals as compared to sailors: it is grossly overweighted with those bearing higher rank in the Civil Service than almost anywhere in the Prison Service. But this, although an extravagance, is not the cause of unrest.

One of the most important tasks that I have to perform as an independent Chief Inspector of Prisons is to promote the appreciation among prison staff that they have a valuable and very difficult role to play in society; and to convey the view to the general public that prisons and those who work in them discharge heavy responsibilities on behalf of the rest of us. In other areas of public life which have similar value to the community, it is not necessary to make the point so often. Although in England we appear to be too ready to minimize the status of many groups of valuable workers – social workers and teachers come to mind – the Prison Service does seem to require particular support. If I am right, that the Prison Service does not enjoy high public regard, I believe that the effects of this bear also upon those specialists who work in prisons, among whom, of course, are prison doctors and medical staff. (I use the word specialist, not in the medical sense, but of someone who works professionally in prison but not in the ordinary Prison Service.)

The prison world is closed in more than one sense. The career route from officer to Governor may follow a number of diverse paths, but the experience gained by an individual, and the recognition of that experience, will come primarily from his or her peer group. In this way, mainstream staff in prisons differ from their specialist colleagues.

The specialist worker within the prison comes from outside with a professional identity created elsewhere. Training and experience as a teacher, doctor or psychologist, start in the profession, through educational institutions which are, of course, part of the community and are only later applied to the prison context. I believe that the source of tension between specialists and main grade staff, is partly to be found in the difference between the career structures of the individuals concerned. Add to this the fact that prison staff routinely work with inmates, whereas some specialist staff come in to provide services, then depart, and it is possible to understand the often expressed view of the prison officer that 'they cannot know what it is *really* like'.

In the past few years efforts have been made to integrate the

Prison Service into the wider community, through the development of such ideas as the community prison, prison open days, and work programmes for prisoners within the community. The *Woolf Report* stated (as I have already set out) that the expectation is that medical treatment for inmates should be of the same standard as the ordinary population would receive on the National Health Service. The report also made clear that the standard of medical care on offer in prison establishments frequently failed to reach this level.

Far-reaching changes in the ways in which prisons are run reached a new stage on 1 April 1993 when the Prison Service became an Executive Agency. Within this structure, medical services will now be provided by the Prison Health Care Services: but health care in prisons remains very much in the Prison Service structure. It does present problems, as I noted in my Annual Report from which I have already quoted another passage:

> Prison medical services appear to remain largely uncoordinated. Some establishments still have unused hospital accommodation and under-employed staff whilst others struggle even to ensure that all inmates are medically screened, however briefly, on reception. Advisory health programmes are virtually non-existent. We must press again for regular medical and dental checkups for lifers and long-termers, and for blood pressure and urine testing as part of a reception screening process which also includes a confidential interview with the doctor who will be responsible for the inmates' ongoing health care. (*Annual Report April 1991 – March 1992*, para 4.93)

Few would doubt that there is room for improvement in prison medical services. The hint in the *Woolf Report* reflects more detailed concerns expressed over many years within the medical profession, by outside commentators and by my own specialist inspectors. Since 1939, many reports have highlighted the problems associated with the provision of medical services in prisons – the *East–Hubert Report* of 1939, the *Gwynne Report* of 1964, the *Butler Report* of 1975, the *Report of the Royal College of Psychiatrists* in 1979 and the 1986 *Report of the Social Services Committee of the House of Commons.* In 1990, the Hoffenberg Working Party brought together the Prison Medical Service and the Royal College of Physicians, and at the same time a Scrutiny of the Prison Medical Service was carried out by the Government Efficiency Unit. Finally, the full report on the training and education of doctors in the Health Care Service for Prisoners prepared by three Royal Colleges, of Physicians, General Practitioners and Psychiatrists, has been published.

Among the suggestions that have been made to improve the

situation are that medical services in prisons should be provided by the NHS, bought in in the same way that probation and education services are at present; a second suggestion has been that prison medicine should be seen as a medical specialty, with practitioners specially trained for the role. I think that both these ideas have merit, but that they do not fully address the problems posed by the practice of medicine in prisons. I would like to use both ideas as the basis for an alternative suggestion.

A large number of small, or low security, prison establishments have had medical services provided by doctors from the NHS (normally General Practitioners providing a number of sessions in each week) for many years. The problem centres on large prisons which require a full-time medical staff. The attraction of the hand-over of such complex closed establishments to the already beleaguered NHS is, I believe, limited. Although many hospital Trusts would like to provide the service, costs have so far been prohibitive. No one is suggesting that prison medicine can be a medical speciality, in the same way as oncology, cardiology or orthopaedics, but it is specialized insofar as it requires knowledge of public health and prison administrative matters which the General Practitioner would not need. Prisoners are members of the general population in particular circumstances. The medical services required, therefore, are the services required by the general population, with the addition of particular links with psychiatric and forensic services which form part of the additional responsibilities of the Head of Medical Services in a prison. The Head of Medical Services, therefore, acts primarily as a General Practitioner and in this capacity should be the first port of call for someone who is sick. This general practice role is supported by many of the recently published reports on prison medicine.

Having said this, I believe that prison populations are worthy of specialist study within the general practice subject area. There is a need for systematic work to be undertaken on the sociomedical characteristics of the prison population, as well as on specifically medical questions relating to the presentation and treatment of illness in the prison environment. I think that it would be helpful for the Prison Health Service to encourage links with Departments of Community Medicine and Public Health to further work on the social aspects of prison medicine and for the general practice area of medicine in prison to be recognized as an area requiring some special training by the three Royal Colleges. This training should be subject to review and accreditation by the Royal Colleges. It is a welcome fact that three Royal Colleges have co-operatively examined prison medical issues, and we must look to their recommendations as to the most appropriate means of preparing doctors for work in the prison context. There is no doubt in my mind that doctors who work full-time in prisons require regular and mandatory access to training programmes which not only update and extend knowledge about issues pertinent to the practice of medicine in prisons; but which also bring the prison doctor into contact with medical colleagues working in other areas of medicine. There is a status issue here which needs to be addressed. Prison doctors must be able to earn professional status equivalent to their colleagues. This is not difficult for those part-time prison medical officers who also work in general practice. It is more difficult for the full-time medical officer.

In this way doctors (and other health care staff, such as nurses, for whom similar conditions should apply) would maintain their professional expertise. Professional well-being demands that such contacts are maintained. The closed world of the prison has in the past tended to remove specialists from this contact. The mainstream Prison Service has much to gain, not only in the improvement to specialist services that would result from suggestions that I have made here in respect of medicine; but also it has much to gain from the possible application of such arrangements to the work of mainstream prison staff. Above all, it would provide a sound basis for the provision of real health care for prisoners.

Commentary

Ann Dally Could someone say a few words about the history of the moral panic that has engulfed us in the past week or two about adolescent crime?

Tumim The figures show quite clearly that the number of serious crimes by juveniles has gone down and not up between 1980 and 1990. The Prison Reform Trust has published a very good statistical paper establishing this. There was an extremely sensible piece in *The Times* the other day by Simon Jenkins setting out the whole correct account, as I understand it, of the figures of what has happened. I would not wish to be taken as in any way to criticize the slightest sneeze or cough by Her Majestys Government, but I think that those pieces are worth considering very carefully.

Speaker I am both an ex-jailer and a historian and I have observed a thirty years cyclical basis. The present Home Secretary's reflex reaction is part of his return to the total incarceration of young offenders. Thirty years ago there were the approved schools, the junior detention centres, the senior detention centres, the Borstals: and far from going away from them, Clarke is now representing a return to that model, and last night's speech was just a slight hastening of the process.

Dr Forsythe Reference has been made to the 1860s and the enormous amount of change that was introduced to the prison system in the 1860s when it swung very vigorously and rapidly over to severity – and this was on the basis in part of an increase of robbery in the street. And it was later shown that this alleged increase was completely fictitious and never actually happened. Unfortunately the change of policy had then been introduced and it was too late for everyone concerned.

Sim If you look at the criminological research area, right back to the nineteenth century we see a series of moral panics about youth in general with categories of youth in particular, black youth in the early 1970s for example. And those kinds of moral panics do lead to panic not just in society at large but within those who are responsible for the government of the country, and consequently we see policies developing out of that reaction, which ultimately are detrimental not just to the young people but detrimental to society at large. There is one more thing: the last 10 days or two weeks have also seen a number of reports of the extent of violence in the country, and I don't see the Home Secretary responding, with the same sense of outrage about the harassment of black people and brown people in the country.

Dr Dorothy Speed As prison exists as a judicial sentence would it not be appropriate for the Home Office Prison Department to hand over its executive power to manage prisons to a Ministry of Justice as in other European countries.

Tumim I cannot get excited at change which involves repainting the door. I think there is a case for amalgamating some functions of the Lord Chancellor's Department with some of the functions of the Home Office. The creation of an agency from the first of April will have the effect of distancing medicine from what goes on in the prisons and give another layer between them and the people running it. I think that there is a certain case that the same people should be dealing with the appointment of judges and the working of the criminal justice system, and the Woolf Report did get started a Criminal Justice Council which is chaired by either a judge nominated by a Lord Chief Justice or by the Permanent Secretary of the Home Office, and which has members from different branches of the criminal justice system, meeting several times a year to discuss common problems, and giving information out to each other about the differing aspects. I have a feeling that that committee could be the precursor – whether you call it the Ministry of Justice or not – for bringing different powers together. I think there is a difficulty in calling it the Ministry of Justice: there is a very long history of having a gentleman called the Lord Chancellor and another gentleman called the Home Secretary and so on, and there are word traditions which should not be lightly disregarded, but getting the functions together is what you are talking about; we are moving somewhat that way, and on this issue I think the direction is right.

Sim If you talk about the legal aid system there are changes likely to cut a swathe through access to justice for a whole series of groups in this country, and it seems to me that there is a real problem of access to justice for individuals and for society.

Tumim We have a Lord Chancellor for legal aid and the Home Secretary for dealing with the prisons; would it make any difference to have a Ministry of Justice to combine these functions?

Sim I would not necessarily come down on the side of a Ministry of Justice. I would want to unlock the criminal justice system of this country in terms of the appointment of judges, the appointment of magistrates, down to those who sit on various industrial tribunals, and I think that the system needs to be opened up.

Dr Peter Nolan One of the possibilities being put forward at the moment is the privatization of prisons, and presumably that is done for a number of reasons one of which is an attempt to change the management culture, with a view to bettering the service. Now the USA has a history of privatized prisons: is there any evidence to date that a privatized prison can address health care needs better, worse or about the same as a state system?

Shaw It happens that the Prison Reform Trust has made a study of this, and I think that there is no evidence that privatized prisons – as such – have improved health care. There are instances in the United States where health care in particular prisons – for example the Riker's Island complex in New York City – has been handed over to a private non-profit hospital, and this does seem to have made a real improvement. Sometimes in the particular context of the American system, contracting-out of health care services has led to an improvement of what was a very bad situation. But the administrative arrangements and policy climate in America are specific to that country, and you cannot necessarily import ideas like that from the United States into the very different circumstances which apply in Britain.

11

The Lessons of History – Concluding Thoughts on The Health of Prisoners: A Historical Symposium

Stephen Shaw

I present these closing thoughts not as a historian or a physician, but as an activist in the contemporary penal reform movement. In other words, as the very imperfect descendant of those iconic figures John Howard and Elizabeth Fry (and of the many lesser-known figures revealed in the essays in this volume).

At first sight, prison reform in the late twentieth century may seem to have little in common with the eighteenth-century movement described by Roy Porter as being hatched by 'cabals of sheriffs and lords lieutenants and J.P.s'. But if the social standing of the reformers may have deteriorated, many of the tensions and contradictions in prison policy with which we grapple have changed little over the years. The German philosopher Hegel wrote that the lesson of history is that people and governments never learn the lessons of history. Certainly we are no closer to resolving the contradictions between the various purposes of imprisonment. And the health care of prisoners remains the mainstream concern of the prison reform lobby which it has been for the past 200 years.

Indeed, any modern reader of these essays will be struck by the historical continuity of certain themes. I do not mean of course that history simply repeats itself. We no longer have the prison tap supplying alcohol to prisoners (at least not officially). We do not have the treadwheel, the crank, the birch, or bread-and-water diets. A century ago, the issue of the appropriate use of psychotropic medicines did not arise, nor – more positively – did the opportunity of running health education programmes in prison.

The prisons themselves have changed, at least so far as physical conditions are concerned. While the image of the dark, dank, insanitary, inner-city pile still applies to some prisons, millions of pounds are being spent on renovating the penal slums. Moreover, there are now as many new gaols as old ones, and the greatest single category is made up of those converted from other purposes – notably from military camps.

The prisoners themselves have changed. We no longer imprison children as we did routinely in the last century. There has been a very substantial growth in the numbers of long-term prisoners, including over 3,000 life sentence prisoners (more than the rest of Western Europe put together). One male prisoner in every six is now from a minority ethnic background, along with one in four female prisoners. Mental health problems amongst prisoners seem to have grown, and increasing numbers of prisoners have problems associated with the misuse of drugs.

But having said this, the strong impression emerging from these essays is that – as Richard Smith writes – 'prisons change little'. Similarly, comparing Broadmoor in the 1860s with Ashworth in 1991, Louis Blom-Cooper remarks that 'nothing very much has changed'. Blom-Cooper adds that if Sir Thomas Erskine returned 'for a brief look at crime today and the treatment of offenders, much, perhaps too much, would appear familiar to him'. I was reminded of another of Sir Louis's maxims – that penal reform should not be equated with penal progress.

Our prisons are of course the physical repositories of history. We are still using one gaol – Oxford – which can trace its history as a place of confinement back 800 years. The very designs of prisons like Pentonville in London and Strangeways in Manchester are expressions of mid-Victorian social philosophy. Even the street names tell a story. Wormwood Scrubs is sited in Du Cane Road, Brixton in Jebb Avenue, lasting memorials to those officers of the Royal Engineers, Sir Edmund Du Cane and Joshua Jebb, who were both literally and metaphorically the architects of the nineteenth-century prison system.

So what common themes may be identified? First, that prisoners have always been a very vulnerable group, experiencing extremely high sickness rates. No fewer than 10 per cent of the prison population now ask to see the doctor every day. Doubtless this figure reflects, in part, the scarcity of proprietary medicines in prison, and prisoners' understandable desire to break the monotony of prison life with a visit to the health care centre. But the figure is astonishingly high when it is remembered that most prisoners are young men, the group who make the least use of medical facilities in the community.

Related to this has been the concern of prison doctors with alleged malingering by prisoners. Of course, malingering may be a perfectly rational tactic on the part of prisoners. We learn from Alison Liebling and Tony Ward that Victorian prisoners 'would feign insanity, and even attempted suicide, in order to escape the full rigours of the prison regime'. I have no doubt that some prisoners currently prefer a visit to the doctor to a morning of drudgery in a prison workshop. But Joe Sim shows how the obsession with 'shamming' has contributed to doctors' identification with the disciplinary hierarchy of the prison. I hear echoes of this all the time from prison doctors explaining why their caseloads are so high, and in that chilling phrase 'attention-seeking behaviour'.

A third theme is the continuing controversy about the quality of medical care provided in prisons, and prisoners' lack of confidence in their physicians. (Although in saying this, I accept as did Judge Tumim, that in certain respects – daily access, provision of dental services – prisoners currently enjoy rights which are 'more eligible' than those which apply to the majority of our fellow citizens.) In her contribution, Anne Hardy reveals that nineteenth-century medical officers did oppose dietary restrictions and the use of hard labour, just as today the Health Care Service for Prisoners has been arguing for effective (but politically controversial) policies to limit the transmission of HIV such as the provision of condoms and needle- exchange schemes. However, I fear that prisoners' general assessment of prison doctors remains very negative. My own postbag at the Prison Reform Trust reflects this, with complaints about medical treatment featuring very heavily.

I have also been struck most forcefully by how similar the pattern of suicides and suicide prevention is today as it was 100 years ago. Then as now, suicides are more likely amongst prisoners facing trial, amongst first-time offenders, amongst those in their first months in custody and at the beginning of long sentences, amongst those convicted of grave crimes, and amongst young offenders. Then as now (or at least until the beginning of the 1990s), suicide prevention consisted of the use of segregation through the use of strip cells, and a system of special watch or surveillance by prison staff.

Current Prison Service initiatives – which explicitly reject the view that suicide is principally a medical issue – have perhaps not been in place long enough for an assessment of their effectiveness. The growth of Listener schemes (using prisoners to help other prisoners), the involvement of the Samaritans, and an emphasis upon the responsibility of the total institution to care for the most vulnerable, are among the most encouraging aspects of the present prison scene. Regrettably, we have yet to witness an impact on the numbers of prisoners who take their own lives – the suicide rate in prison is now running at roughly one death every eight days.

Other themes also emerge. One is the fear of contagion between prison and the outside world. Is there a parallel here between present concerns about HIV transmission in prisons and the eighteenth-century alarm over so-called gaol fever? Roy Porter says apropos of John Howard that 'typhus proved the best prison reformer'. To date, there are few signs that the AIDS pandemic will exert a similar force for good.

Another common strand is the continuing debate about less eligibility (the assumed requirement that, in no circumstances, should prisoners be treated more favourably than law-abiding members of society). Another is criticism of the quality of management in prisons. Yet another is controversy over the degree to which prison conditions and the fact of imprisonment can aggravate physical and mental ill health.

I note too the conflating of issues of medical and moral health. Two centuries ago, John Howard applied poor medical and hygiene standards as an index of the ability of the prison to act as a reformative institution. I see something very similar in Judge Tumim's many inspection reports today.

Particularly depressing is our seeming inability to meet the needs of prisoners with mental health problems. Anne Hardy tells us that in the nineteenth century 'neither the asylums nor the prisons wanted the responsibility' for criminal lunatics as they were termed. Although I am told that transfers from prison to psychiatric hospital are now more readily agreed than in the 1980s, a recent study by Professor John Gunn and colleagues from the Institute of Psychiatry suggests that well over 1,000 prisoners have mental health problems of sufficient seriousness that they would come within the remit of the Mental Health Act. Any visitor to the unconvicted wing of one of our local prisons will know that large numbers of people in psychiatric distress are still being inappropriately remanded into prison for medical reports. Just as with the criminal lunatics, so neither the Prison Service nor the Health Service seems to want responsibility for offenders with mental health needs.

In tracing these continuities, there are of course still gaps in our knowledge. It would be interesting to know more about the quality and training of prison medical staff over the years, particularly that of paramedical staff. We need to know more too about the links with mainstream health care. And, as Joe Sim makes clear in his typically trenchant contribution, we have only limited knowledge of prisoners' actual experiences, and especially the experiences of women prisoners. Consulting prisoners and taking their views seriously are still in their infancy in the Prison Service, as they are surely in medical practice generally.

Perhaps the most significant continuing theme emerging from these essays has been concern about the dual responsibilities of prison medical officers to prison management and to their prisoner-patients. Martin Wiener outlines this conflict between punishment and care in terms of the balance between the Benthamite principles of lenity, severity and economy. Anne Hardy describes some of the wide range of duties – some to their patients, some to their institution – which were the responsibility of nineteenth-century medical officers, many of which come down to us today in doctors assessing prisoners' 'fitness for work' and 'fitness for punishment'.

This embrace between medicine and discipline in prisons reached its nadir in the medicalizing of control through the use of drugs in the 1960s and 1970s. Prisoners tell me this is far less common today, and that they are as likely now to be denied psychotropic medicines they have been prescribed by their GPs in the community, as they are to be given these drugs inappropriately.

The critical issue is about the self-identification of prison doctors as either personal physicians or as key members of the management of the institution to which they are attached. The conflict is inherent in any closed institution, and affects other prison specialists like psychologists, prison teachers, and probation officers working in prison. But it has been most acute amongst doctors, and seems unlikely to be resolved until either the NHS takes full responsibility for prison health care or (at a minimum) the recommendations of the Efficiency Scrutiny on the Prison Medical Service are fully implemented.

Prison medicine has developed, if not as a specialism, at least as a separate and isolated arm of medicine. There are special responsibilities – managerial, environmental health, report writing – but, as Richard Smith argues, most of these could and should be carried out by someone other than prisoners' personal physicians.

I am, however, encouraged by recent progress within the Health Care Service for Prisoners (a change of name from the Prison Medical Service I regard as more than symbolic). I particularly commend the greater emphasis on preventative services. Nevertheless, the general isolation of prison medicine remains bad for prisoners, and for the professional development of prison doctors. One great advantage of closer integration with the NHS will be that the profession as a whole could better police itself. In arguing that case, I and other contemporary prison reformers will have been greatly helped by the contributions first presented at the Royal Society of Medicine/ Wellcome Institute for the History of Medicine symposium and now reproduced in this volume.

Index

A

Abnett, Thomas *30, 31*
Account of the Principal Lazarettos in Europe *8, 14*
Acheson, Sir Donald *146*
Acland, Henry *64*
Act for the Better Government of Convict Prisons *60*
adolescence and adolescent crime *127, 168*
Afro-Caribbean prisoners *103*
AIDS *174*
alcoholism *126, 138, 143*
American Independence *15*
amputations *67*
apothecary *7, 28, 30, 32–5, 39, 87*
arson *121*
Ashworth Hospital *157, 158*
Ashworth Inquiry *160*
Askham, Henry Francis *61, 76, 81*
assaults on prison staff *73*
Association for the Improvement of Women Prisoners in Newgate *84*
audit *143*
authoritarianism *75*
Aylesbury Female Convict Prison *61*

B

Baly, William *62, 71*
Barlinnie Prison *140*
Bauman, Zygmunt *103*
Baumgartner, Leona *6*
Bedford, Duchess of *111*
beer supply *37*
Bentham, Jeremy *15, 44, 45, 55, 137*
Benthamism *44–58*
  two faces of *49*
  'Victorian' elements of *46*
Bethlem Hospital *154*
biometrics *127*
Blackburn, William *9*
Blaker, E.S. *67, 76*
Blom-Cooper, Sir Louis *172*
Board of Health *49*
Borstal system *127*
Botanic Garden *5*
Bowles, William Leslie *5*
Boynton Report *160*
Bradley, Charles Lawrence *61*
British Ladies' Society for Promoting the Reformation of Female Prisoners *83, 84, 87, 90, 91, 94, 96, 97*
British Medical Journal *143*
Brixton Prison *65, 73, 94*
Broadmoor Hospital *151–62*
  creation of *155–6*
  full capacity *158*
  management *157*
Brockway, Fenner *107, 108*
Brown, James Baldwin *5*
bubonic plague *14*
Bull, Lady Megan *138*
Burns, John *61, 66*
Butler Committee on Mentally Abnormal Offenders *160*
Butler Report *160, 165*
Buxton, Sir Thomas Fowell *85*

C

Calderstones Asylum *107*
Campbell, John *71*
capstan *70*
Cardiff Prison *131*
Carlyle, Thomas *6*
Carnarvon Committee on Prisons *52, 53, 64, 65, 68*
Carter, Charles *110*
Chadwick, Edwin *49, 50, 51, 55*
chaplains *39, 94, 124–6*
charity boxes *29*
Chatham Prison *61, 65, 66, 68*

Chief Inspector of Prisons *164*
children in prison *143*
Christie, Nils *103*
Clarke, Kenneth *149, 168*
Clarke, Vans Christian *61, 64, 69*
Clerkenwell Prison *124*
Coke *153*
Coldbath Fields House of Correction *89*
colic *66*
Commission on Criminal Lunacy *72, 74*
Commissioners in Lunacy *156*
Committee of Scientific Inquiry *65*
Committee on Prison Dietaries *52*
Committee on the Prisons of the Metropolis *86*
condoms distribution *143, 173*
Conolly, John *157*
Cook, James *11*
copy-cat effect *132, 133*
Corne, Rev. William *30*
County Gaol *27*
crank *70*
Crawford, William *89*
Criminal Justice Act *102, 110*
Criminal Lunacy Commission *72, 74*
criminal lunatic asylum system *151–62*
criminal lunatics *73, 154, 159, 174*
Criminal Lunatics Act 1800 *154*
criminality
  and mental health *93*
  theories *109*
Crofton, Sir Walter *68*
Crowthorne's disease *154, 158, 160*
cruelty in prisons *115, 123*
Crutchley, Brooks *33, 34*
Cullen, M.J. *44*
cultural change *142*

D

Dadd, Richard *155*
dangerous lunatics *154*
dangerous prisoners *136, 151*
Dartmoor Prison *60, 71, 72*
Darwin, Erasmus *5*
Davenhill, Ann *28*
death sentence *39*
deaths *54, 103, 111, 125*
  see also suicide
debtor prisoners *29, 31, 36, 39*
debtors' ward *9*
DeLacy, Margaret *14, 15, 16*
delinquents *46, 127*
Departmental Commission on Criminal Lunacy *62–3*
depression *123, 131*
deterrence *47*
diabetes *140*
dietary management *28, 33, 36, 52, 53, 65–68, 75, 86, 88, 90, 103, 110, 122, 173*
dignity *147*
Directors of Convict Prisons *67*
Discharged Prisoners' Aid Society *94*
disciplinary technologies *16*
district health authorities *142*
district visiting movement *91*
Dixon, Hepworth *5, 8*
Dolphin, Henry *32*
Donkin, Horatio *106*
drug problems *140, 143*
Du Cane, Sir Edmund *122, 172*
dungeons *36*

E

East, Norbert *137*
East, Norwood *106*
East, W. Norwood *126*
East-Hubert Report *165*
electroconvulsive therapy *110*
Elizabeth Fry Refuge *84, 90*
emotional instability *126, 127*
English Convict, The *121*
English Prisons Today *107*
Enlightenment *5, 103*
environmental factors *127*
epidemics *16*
epilepsy *72, 126*
Erskine, Sir Thomas *153, 172*
ethical issues *112*
ethnic backgrounds *172*

Evils of England Social and Economic, The 63
Executive Agency *165*

F

family health service authorities *142*
Farr, William *49, 50, 55*
fear *123, 124*
feeble-minded prisoners *126*
feeding *see* dietary management
Feltham *127*
female prisoners *see* women prisoners
Festina Lente *154*
fevers *11*
Fieldhouse *34*
fitness for punishment *175*
fitness for work *175*
food *see* dietary management
force-feeding *112, 141*
Foucault, Michel *46, 48, 103, 104, 136*
Four Stages of Cruelty *115*
Frazer, Catherine *95*
Fry, Elizabeth *83–101, 132, 137, 171*

G

gaol distemper *33, 35*
gaol fever *10, 12–15, 34, 174*
gaol keepers *48*
Gaol Visiting Guide *87*
gaolers *7, 27, 28, 30–4, 36, 37, 39*
Garland, David *106*
general practitioners *140, 166*
George III *38*
Gill, Dr *107*
Gladstone Committee on Prisons *55, 69, 105, 135, 137*
Gladstone Report *102*
Glancy report *160*
Good, John Mason *9*
Gordon, Mary *112*
Goring, Charles *121*
Gover, Robert M. *62, 69, 70, 75, 81, 105, 119, 120, 122–6*
Government Efficiency Unit *165*
governors *37, 125, 147, 148*
Grant, Helen *90*
Grave of Howard, The *5*
Greenhow, Headlam *67*
Grellet, Stephen *84, 85*
Grey, Sir George *94*
Gunn, John *174*
Gurney, John Joseph *85, 89, 91*
Guy, William Augustus *51–5, 62–5, 67–76, 96*
Gwynne Report *165*

H

Habermas, Jurgen *103*
Hadfield *38*
Hale *153*
Hales, Stephen *15*
Halevy, Elie *44*
Hall, Gillian *107*
Haller, Dr *12*
Hamilton, David *66*
Harcourt, Henry *69, 122*
hard labour *68, 69, 76, 173*
Hare, David *136*
Hastings, G.W. *70*
Hatfield, James *153*
Hayley, William *5*
Head of Medical Services *166*
Health Care Service for Prisoners *164, 175*
health care services *48, 49, 53, 102–17, 165, 173*
  commentary *146–50*
  purchasing of *142, 147, 148*
health of prisoners *10, 11, 44–58, 71, 87, 142*
Health of Prisoners Act *7, 59*
Health of Towns Association *51*
Health Service for Prisoners *134–50*
health standards *7*
health status *147*
heart disease *75*
Helps, Dr *154*
Herbert, Sidney *95*
High Security Working Group *161*
Himmelfarb, Gertrude *46*
HIV infection *142, 173, 174*

Hoare, Samuel *85*
Hobhouse, Stephen *107, 108*
Hoffenberg Working Party *165*
Hogarth *116*
Holloway Prison *108, 111, 138*
Home Office *106, 125, 137, 138, 142, 144, 157–9*
Home Office Efficiency Scrutiny *141–2*
homicide *151*
Hopkins, Gerard Manley *91*
Horsley, John *124*
hospital block *147*
Hospital Trusts *166*
Houghton, William *65, 66*
Houses of Correction *27, 29, 30, 36, 38*
Howard Association *94*
Howard, John *5–26, 35, 36, 51, 54, 86, 171*
  Bedfordshire estate *11–12*
  birth *6*
  commentary *25–6*
  death *5, 16*
  expeditions at home and abroad *7*
  High Sheriff of Bedfordshire *7*
  'imagining the penitentiary' *11*
  imprisonment *6*
  interest in medicine *12*
  life style *8*
  prison expert *7*
Howard medal *52*
Hubert, W.H. de B. *137*
Hughes, Francis *34, 37*
Hughes, Richard *34, 35*
Hughes, Robert *34*
humane containment *138*
humanitarianism *75*
Humby, William *89*
hunger strikes *141*
hygiene *110–11, 174*

I

imprisonment
  purposes of *135–6, 144, 171*
  see also prisons
impulsiveness *126*
infliction of pain *47*
inquests *125*
Insane in Private Dwellings, The *74*
insanity *38, 71, 72, 75, 124–6, 151, 173*
Irish prisoners *116*

J

Jarvis, John *30*
Jebb, Sir Joshua *64, 92, 93, 172*
Jenkins, Simon *168*
Johnston, Valerie *66*
Journal of the Statistical Society *51*
juvenile crime *168*

K

Keeper of the County Gaol *27*
Knight, Philip *131*

L

lady visitors *87, 88, 91, 94, 96*
Lady Visitors' Association *94*
Lamb, Charles *5, 6*
Lancaster, Edwin *82*
Lancet, The *49, 64, 67*
Lee, Francis *30, 31*
legal aid system *169*
lessons of history *171–6*
leucotomy *110*
Liebling, Alison *118, 173*
life sentence prisoners *172*
Lind, James *11*
Linebaug, Peter *116*
listener schemes *131, 132, 173*
London Hanged, The *116*
long-term prisoners *172*
Lunacy Commissioners' Report *158*
lunatic asylums *11*
lunatics *38*
Lunatics Act of 1845 *155*
Lunatics Act of 1860 *155*
Lushington, Sir Godfrey *138*
Lytton, Constance *112*

M

Macartney, Wilfred *108*
McCullough, Dr *159*
MacDonagh, Oliver *16*

McNaughton, Daniel *154–5*
Maitland, Dr *64*
malingering by prisoners *76, 124, 172–3*
maltreatment allegations *160*
management *147–8, 169, 174*
  problems *146*
  responsibilities *141*
  see also dietary management
Master of the House of Correction *27*
matron *84, 89*
May Committee *138, 139*
Maybrick, Florence *111, 112*
Mead, Richard *15*
mechanical restraint *109*
Medical Act 1858 *59*
medical examinations *112*
Medical Inspector of Local Prisons *61*
medical officers *60, 61, 75–6*
medical training programmes *166–7*
medical treatment *39*
Memoir of the Public and Private Life of John Howard, Philanthropist *5*
menstruation *112*
mental cases *71, 73*
Mental Defectives Act 1913 *126*
Mental Deficiency Act 1913 *106, 158*
mental health *11, 92, 106, 124, 172, 174*
  and criminality *93*
Mental Health Act *159, 174*
Mental Health Act Commission *157, 159*
mentally abnormal offenders *151–62*
Meredith, Susanna *94*
Metropolitan Commissioners in Lunacy *155*
Meyer, Dr *156, 157*
midwife *28*
Millbank Penitentiary *81*
Millbank Prison *51, 60, 62, 65, 72, 94–6, 122*
Mitchell, Arthur *74*
moral health *174*
Morris, Norval *138*
Moss Side *158–9*
Mothercraft *113*
mothers and babies *143*
'Murmuring Judges' *136*

N

National Association for the Promotion of Social Science *95*
National Association of Prison Visitors *94*
National Association of Visitors to Women Prisoners *94*
National Health Act of 1977 *159*
National Health Service Act of 1946 *159*
National Health Service (NHS) *102, 108, 141, 142, 144, 146, 147, 149, 150, 163, 165, 166, 175*
necrosis *67*
needle-exchange schemes *173*
Neild, James *9*
Newgate Prison *15, 84, 89, 91*
Nicholson, Margaret *154*
Nightingale, Florence *95, 98*
Nightingale Training School *97*
normalization *140*
Northallerton Prison *70*
Norwich Prison *120*
nursing reform *91*
nutrition *65–7*
  see also dietary management

O

O'Brien, Captain D. *96*
Observations on the Visiting, Superintendence and Government of Female Prisons *97*
Ode to Howard *5*
offences *contra naturam* *72*
Oglethorpe *15*
O'Malley, Susan *107*
Orange, Dr *73*
Orr, Jim *140*
overcrowding *15–16*
Oxford Prison *172*

P

Pailthorpe, Grace *113*
Panopticon prison plan *45, 46*
paramedical staff *174*

Park Lane *158, 160*
Parkhurst Prison *60, 65, 72*
parole board reports *141*
Paul, Sir George Onesiphorus *15*
pauper lunatics *154*
Peel, Sir Robert *59, 92, 155*
penal Benthamism *45, 46, 48*
Penal Discipline *112*
Penal Practice in a Changing Society (White paper) *137*
Penal Servitude Commission *68*
Penitentiary Houses *36*
Pentonville Prison *60, 61, 65, 92, 127, 172*
Percy Commission *159*
physical health *92*
Pickering, Ian *139*
Pilling, Joe *163*
planning of prisons *9*
political deviants *116*
Poor Law Board *68*
Poor Laws *116*
Popham, Alexander *35*
Portland Prison *60, 65, 66, 68, 76*
Powell, Enoch *159*
pregnant women *112*
Preston Prison *125*
preventable injury or illness *47*
preventative services *140*
Prevention of Crime Act 1908 *125*
preventive philanthropy *52*
Pringle, Sir John *11, 15*
Prison Act of 1865 *70*
Prison Act of 1877 *70*
Prison Act of 1898 *106*
prison administration *7, 10*
prison cells *38*
Prison Commissioners *70, 127*
prison conditions *9–10, 13, 15, 46, 107, 110–11, 134, 135, 171–2*
prison doctors *102, 167*
prison hospitals *66, 76*
Prison Medical Reform Council (PMRC) *108, 112*
Prison Medical Service *59–80, 102–17*
  commentary *81–2*
  mission statement *135*
  role of *135*
  see also Health Service for Prisoners
Prison Officers Association *160*
prison reform *5, 12, 14–16, 138, 141, 171*
Prison Reform Trust *168, 170, 173*
Prison System Enquiry Committee *112*
prison visitors *87, 94*
  see also lady visitors
prisoners' rights organizations *108*
prisons
  aims of *139*
  planning *9*
  positive role of *137*
  sanitary state *7*
  see also imprisonment
Prisons Act 1865 *59*
Prisons for Women: Some Accounts of Life in Holloway *112*
privatization of prisons *170*
Probation of Offenders Act 1907 *125*
Prole, John *7*
Prout, Curtis *55*
psychiatry *106, 109–11, 113, 118, 131*
psychological health *109*
psychological testing *113*
psychological treatments *137, 140*
psychotherapy *137, 138*
psychotropic drugs *103, 110*
public health services *6, 53, 141*
punishment *47, 52–5, 68, 75, 76, 91, 96, 109, 112, 113, 123, 135, 137, 139, 141*
purchasing of health care *142, 147, 148*
Purioll, Phillip *31*

Q

Quakers *110*
  see also Fry, Elizabeth

R

racial discrimination *116*
Rampton Hospital *158, 160*
rape *72*
rations *66*
recidivists *136*

reconviction rates *136*
Red Collar Man *108*
Reed Committee *161*
Reed, John *161*
Rees, Merlyn *5*
regional secure units *160*
rehabilitation *137–8, 141, 149*
remorse *124*
Rendle, J.D. *61*
Report of the Royal College of Psychiatrists *165*
Report of the Social Services Committee of the House of Commons *165*
Report on the Sanitary Condition of the Labouring Population *49*
reports for courts and parole board *141*
research *143, 168*
Richardson, Benjamin Ward *59*
Robbins, William *32*
rogues *38*
Rolle, John Denny *9–10*
Rollin, Henry *154*
Royal Commission into Sterilization *107*
Royal Commission on Penal Servitude *62, 65, 67, 76, 96, 122*
Royal Commission on the Care and Control of the Feeble-Minded *106*
rule of economy *48*
rule of lenity *47, 48*
rule of severity *47, 48*
Russell, Rev. Whitworth *89*

S

Samaritans *131, 173*
sanitary arrangements *39*
scientific humanitarianism *52*
Scott, Peter *151*
scrofula *65*
Scrutiny on the Prison Medical Service *163, 165*
scurvy *11, 16*
Second World War *108*
security considerations *136, 139, 152, 160*
self-respect *147*
Senior, Nassau *46*
sentencing criteria *88*
separate confinement *71, 92*
sex offenders *140, 143*
shame *124*
shamming test *107–8*
Sharpey, William *64*
sheriff *27*
shot-drill *70*
sickness rates *172*
Sim, Joe *60, 122, 173*
Smalley, Dr *106, 107, 125–7*
Smalley, Sir Herbert *120, 121*
smallpox *14*
Smith, Edward *64*
Smith, Richard *60, 149*
Snails Progress *110*
social discipline *105–9*
social reconstructionist ideology *109*
Society for the Improvement of Prison Discipline *85*
Society for the Propagation of Christian Knowledge *15*
solitary confinement *91, 93, 107, 108*
soup-kitchen philanthropy *63*
Special Hospital Service Authority *159*
Special Hospitals *152, 159–62*
specialist medical services *140*
Spierenberg, Peter *9*
spirituous liquors *37*
Stafford Gaol *27–43*
State of the Prisons in England and Wales, The *7, 9–12, 35*
Statistical Society *51*
Strahan, S.A.K. *121*
Strangeways Prison *125, 172*
strip cells *142, 173*
suicide *118–33, 142, 173, 174*
  attempted *130*
  causes of *126*
  commentary *130–3*
  early studies *119–25*
  motives for *125*
  prevention *128, 130*
  reasons for *122*
  survey *119*
Suicide and Insanity *121*

Sullivan, Ellen *111*
Superintending Medical Officer of Convict Prisons *61*
surgeons *7, 28, 30, 31, 34, 35, 37, 39*

T

taskmaster *39*
Thompson, Edith *112*
Thorley, Edward *32*
Thornton, Dr *105*
training
 medical programmes *166–7*
 women prisoners *113*
training and treatment of convicted prisoners *138–9*
transportation *36*
treadmill *68–70, 75, 87, 89*
treatment
 consent *143*
 model *139*
 of convicted prisoners *138–9*
 vs. punishment *137*
tuberculosis *65*
Twining, Louisa *98*
typhus *6, 11, 16, 174*

U

ulcer cases *76*
Utilitarianism *44–7, 52*

V

vagabonds *38*
Vagrancy Act of 1714 *152*
Vagrancy Act of 1744 *152*
Verses to John Howard 5
violence *72*

W

Wakefield Prison *125*
Walker, George *61*
Walton Prison *117*
War of Independence *35*
Ward, John *34*
Ward, Tony *173*
weak-minded prisoners *71–5*
Wedgewood, John *30, 31*
Wetwood, Job *32, 33*
Wiener, Martin *106*
Willan, Robert *85*
wine supplies *37*
Woking Prison *73, 111*
women prisoners *36, 39, 84, 103, 108, 111–13, 138, 143, 172*
 training *113*
Woolf Committee *134*
Woolf Report *132–3, 139, 163–70*
Wormwood Scrubs Prison *61, 137, 172*
Wormwood Scrubs Prison Annexe *140*
Wrench, Matilda *91, 97*
Wright, Thomas *34*

Y

young offenders *127*
Young, Peter *105*